Contents

chapter one

the shape we're in

We're overweight; we're underweight. **We aren't exercising enough;** we're addicted to exercise. **We're pumping ourselves full of overprocessed, fatty and additive-high junk food;** we'll eat only organic foods. **We're couch potatoes who watch too much TV;** we never sit still and relax. **We're drinking too much alcohol, sugary fizzy drinks and caffeine;** we'll touch only designer bottled waters flown thousands of miles from a Pacific outpost.

We've never had it so good; we've never been more stressed out. We are surrounded by abundance; we are surrounded by temptation. We're living longer than ever before and enjoying safer and more comfortable lives and better health, yet we've never been more worried about our health and our looks. Never have we been more focused on our bodies. One minute we are reading reports about how we're living much longer and the next we are in the middle of an epidemic of heart disease and cancer. And almost every week new scientific reports come out, often seemingly contradictory.

Let me tell you what I want. I want everyone to start leading healthier, happier lives. And here's the secret: one of the best ways I know to enjoy life and be healthy is to eat well and enjoy your food.

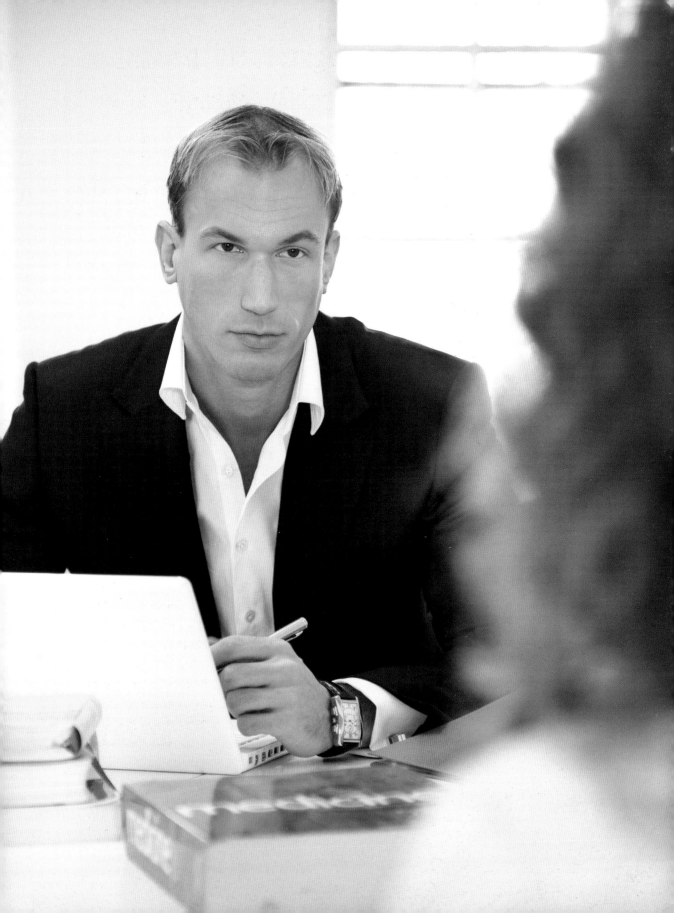

But aren't we getting too **fat?**

In the UK it is estimated that around 30,000 deaths a year occur because of complications resulting from obesity. Around 2.6 million people in the UK live with the effects of heart conditions, with about 600,000 deaths a year as a result. Billions of pounds are spent by the National Health Service treating heart disease but a much smaller amount on preventing it in the first place. The blame for most of these deaths can be laid at the door of unhealthy lifestyle choices including smoking, bad eating patterns and a lack of exercise. The information on how to live healthily is out there and available, but are we really listening, or are we simply being confused by the pages of nonsense that are being peddled as fact?

Currently, 10 per cent of six-year-olds are classified as 'obese' and 17 per cent of 15-year-olds. Almost a quarter of UK citizens are technically obese, and a mind-numbing three-quarters are officially overweight. Experts predict that by 2020, if we continue to grow as we are doing, a third of British adults and half of British children will be obese. (See page 33 for the official definitions of overweight and obesity.)

On top of all of this, we are undeniably passing poor lifestyle habits on to our children. Official figures for 1995 to 2004 show that the number of dangerously overweight children (11–15 years old) has risen to around 25 per cent. We do everything in our power to protect and love our children yet are unwittingly condemning them to a life of health problems. Politicians are fond of promising us ever-increasing life choices, but when it comes to our diet we could be killing ourselves and our children with kindness.

Up to half a century ago, home-makers would spend three to four hours each day washing, cleaning and beating carpets, and the farmers among us – a much more common profession in the past than it is now – would work all day tilling the fields, milking the cows and harvesting crops. It was hard work and required a lot of energy. Now we have machines to do much of this for us, but the exercise we got doing these labour-intensive and boring tasks has not always been replaced by something else. Instead it takes us a few hours a week at most to fill a shopping trolley, that is, if we are not doing our food shopping online. We don't even have to expend energy carrying heavy bags home. The most we do, if we're not getting it delivered to our door, is load it up in the car. The hard graft of our grandparents and beyond may have been monotonous and boring, but our less active lifestyle could be harming us.

Faced with an incredible array of foods to choose from, we're also making some poor diet decisions. With two world wars during the first half of the last century, most people's concern was getting enough to eat. The peace and prosperity of the subsequent years have led to a plentiful supply of food, which in turn has brought concerns about our eating habits that have never occurred before. We are suffering from what has been termed 'a malnutrition of affluence'.

Over the past few years, portion sizes in restaurants, bistros and takeaways have been gradually getting bigger, and this trend is causing concern among health professionals. It's one of the ways in which we might be eating more than we need.

Food **revolution**

The last few decades in the western world have seen huge advancements in food production and distribution. We can have any food flown over to our country round the clock. So what we want, we get – any time of the year. Supermarkets and food manufacturers have growing numbers of development departments conjuring up all sorts of new foods that only need to be shoved into a hot oven or microwave for a few minutes. Many will have flashes on the front of their packs claiming they are reduced fat and included in their so-called 'healthy eating' range.

Low-down

Retailers are stocking an increasing range of low-fat foods. However, be sure to read the label. There are two things to be aware of. To use the term 'fat-reduced' on a product, the manufacturer only has to reduce the fat by 25 per cent, and if the fat content was very high in the first place, you won't be much better off. Secondly, the fat reduction might have been achieved with the addition of something else, such as extra sugar. Vegetarians should also check the ingredients lists, as gelatine is sometimes added to foods as a thickener to take the place of some of the fat.

Dieting to lose weight is, as we shall see, in historical terms a fairly recent phenomenon, and it is tied in to the rise of our consumption of low-cost processed foods, especially takeaway fast foods. It is easy to mince meat to turn into burgers so they cook quickly on a griddle. Potatoes are cut into even-size sticks and deep-fried because it is quicker than boiling or mashing. They can be fat-blanched, frozen and when ready to serve, tipped into a deep-fat fryer full of hot oil to brown and crisp. With the rise in fast-food outlets has come a rise in obesity and health problems associated with a high-fat, low-exercise lifestyle.

Advances in fast-food management and the entry of creative chefs into the mass-market food business are beginning to see the launch of successful healthier fast-food outlets selling freshly prepared healthy salads wraps, falafels, soups, griddled chicken and tuna with a Mediterranean/Californian twist, such as the Leon chain. Not a moment too soon.

Or are we
wasting away?

At the other end of the scale, all is not well either. An increasing number of us are underweight because we are deliberately undereating, for a variety of psychological and emotional reasons.

B-eat (the eating disorders charity) estimates around 90,000 Britons are receiving treatment for anorexia and bulimia, and that figure doesn't take into account sufferers who haven't come forward for any help or don't think they have a problem. The tragedy is the high death rate, accounting for up to 20 per cent of deaths from psychiatric conditions.

Eating disorders are responsible for more loss of life than any other psychological illness. Many sufferers are in the vulnerable 14—25 year age group and most are female, although the number of male sufferers is rising.

Behind every eating disorder statistic is a human story of anxiety, lack of self-esteem and depression. Some of these cases could be avoided, or at least eased, especially in the early stages, by making simple changes to a healthier eating pattern. Those with acute psychological disorders need to seek medical help and counselling, but if families and friends of those who are in danger of developing these disorders are encouraged to talk openly with their loved ones (especially teenagers going through puberty) and helped with information and advice, they might be able to steer sufferers away from dangerous eating patterns before they take hold.

The history of slim

More than three-quarters of women equate being slim with being happy. The obsession with slim, however, is relatively new.

Historically, women's ideal body shape has been associated with fecundity. Ancient statues and figurines of goddesses show them with generous bottoms and rolls of frontal fat, conditions that would now shoot them into the overweight super league. Not so much survival of the fittest, but the fattest. Seventeenth-century paintings show female models with voluptuous curves caressing cherubic children plump and pink with chubby arms and rolls of soft fat. Fatness was seen as a sign of plenty and contentment. Even scantily clothed nymphs had rounded tummies and bottoms.

The Victorians admired women with well-covered, sloping shoulders tapering to a tiny, nipped-in waist. Whalebone corsets encased and enhanced natural curves, sometimes to the extent of putting pressure on internal organs. The rising emancipation of women during and after the First World War freed them from the constraints of tight clothing and by the 1920s and 1930s fashion houses began to produce lighter clothes following more natural lines. But it meant there were no longer any frills or flounces for women to hide behind. Their bodies were on display with all their little imperfections.

The 1950s saw the launch of the bikini, and suddenly women had the chance to expose bare midriffs. But 1950s women were still mostly 'nicely covered'. Marilyn Monroe, a healthy size 14, remains an icon 50 years after her death, but her figure is no longer the ideal to which we aspire.

In the 1960s, fashions became skimpier and ideal body shapes thinner. Plump teenage girls were told they would soon grow out of their puppy fat. Many didn't and they suffered agonies of self-consciousness. It was around this part of the 20th century that dieting started to become big business, with magazines beginning the now familiar seasonal diet features to 'help' their readers.

And somehow the obsession with dieting, far from going away, gradually became more entrenched.

Celebrity role models

Now, our fascination with celebrities drives the media to delve into every aspect of their lives, particularly their body shapes, on which they are increasingly judged. Magazine front covers send out mixed messages, one week claiming certain actresses or soap stars are worryingly thin and the next flashing straplines of 'spot the cellulite' on the photos of some hapless star's thighs as she clambers out of a car in the tiniest skirt. Male stars are not exempt. They are snapped with a telescopic lens as they stroll on a beach showing a nice rounded paunch. It seems that we relish these details, perhaps because they bring the celebrities down from their pedestals and make them seem 'more like us'.

Sometimes a magazine will carry both messages in one issue: what is worse, bony shoulders or dimpled thighs? New celebrity mums are applauded for getting back into shape within weeks of giving birth, following a strict diet and exhausting exercise regime. And other new mums want to follow them. Except they don't have access to the personal dieticians and trainers (not to mention live-in nannies to mind the baby), so they embark on a more homespun regime: they just stop eating.

Any celebrity star who starts as 'nicely covered' and proud of it, within a year or two falls into the diet trap and gets praised in glamour magazines for looking 'stunning'. She's joined the size 10 set. We judge our female celebrities by their dress sizes. Sizes 8 to 10 are now seen as normal, while size 16 is not. Yet most women in the UK are a 14 or 16. That means that in reality sizes 14 and 16 are the norm – they are normal. Our perceptions of normal have become skewed.

Girls want taut stomachs, but the female stomach is not naturally taut. The belly has to be soft enough to expand during pregnancy. Bums and breasts are supposed to be rounded and developed. Young female celebrities get thinner and thinner, lose their natural curves and then end up undergoing surgery to implant what nature had given them to begin with.

If we are to be happy and healthy we need to understand our bodies, find our ideal weight and then maintain our physique by enjoyable exercise and eating a nutritious and balanced diet.

The statue of David

Fashions for the perfect female body shape have varied over the centuries but for us men it is a much simpler story. Michelangelo's 500-year-old statue of David in Florence with its perfect six-pack stomach, slim hips and firm rippling chest is still seen as the perfect representation of the male physique. Within reason, the fitter and stronger we are, the better we look. But look a little closer at this great work of art. You can see that the head and upper body of David are too large for the rest of his body, and that his right hand is also disproportionately big. He has been sculpted this way deliberately so that when he is viewed from below he seems the image of male perfection that we still subscribe to today. To achieve this apparent perfection, the artist deliberately distorted the image. The desired look is one that does not exist in reality – and this is the case with many of the images of 'perfection' we are presented with and strive to attain.

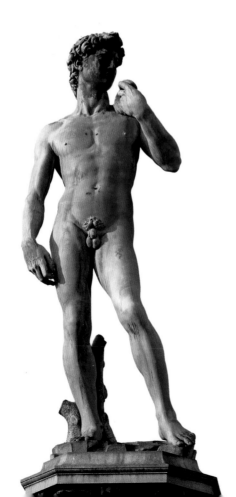

If Barbie
were lifesize

She'd probably be 1.75 metres (5 foot 9 inches) tall and weigh about 47 kilos (7½ stone). With such a low body weight, her periods would probably stop. Her measurements would most likely be 39–18–33, and she would look like a freak. It's not just girls who are presented with unattainable 'ideals' in childhood. I had an action figure called GI Joe. If GI Joe were lifesize, he'd probably have a 140cm (55-inch) chest and 70cm (27-inch) biceps, which would make his arms almost as big as his waist. No competitive body builder achieves these kinds of dimensions.

It's about diet, not dieting.

chapter two

our emotional relationship with food

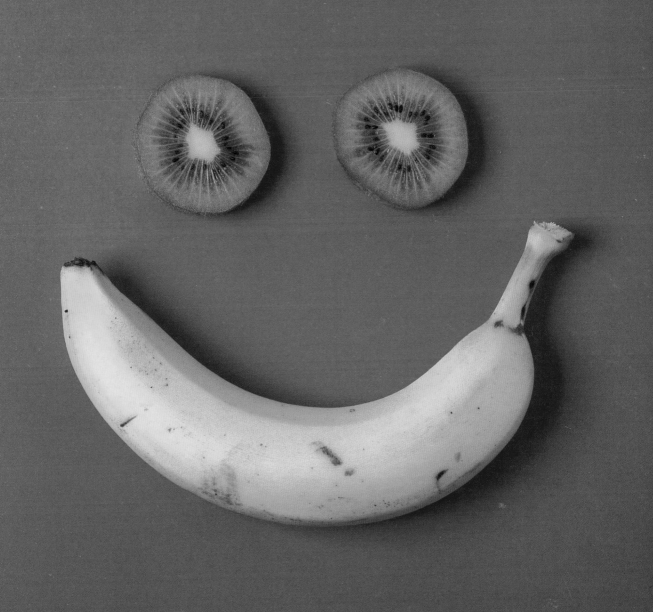

We need food to function. Our body tells us when we need to eat. **Lucky us: there's plenty of food about. It's all quite simple, really. So why has it become so complicated? Why do we sometimes eat according to how we feel, even when that feeling is not hunger?** And why is our response to how we feel sometimes not to eat at all, even when we are hungry?

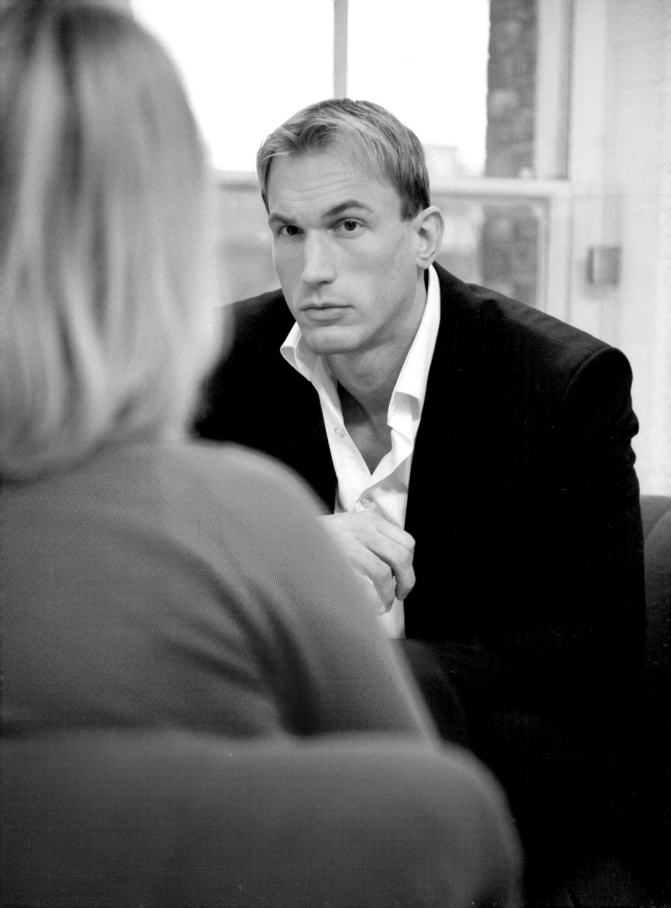

Feeling good,
feeling bad

We eat for many reasons. First and most basic, we eat to stay alive. Our food is our fuel. We need air, water and food – the basics without which we would die. Our need for fuel is powerful; it's a strong drive that's hard to ignore. It's there to ensure our survival. However, eating is a source of pleasure, too. There's a reason for this. The pleasure we get from eating is a secondary drive, helping to ensure we continue to seek out food, even in the face of danger and difficulty, and providing reward for our efforts. Pleasure also supplies us with a clue as to the suitability of the foods we choose: poisonous foods generally taste bitter or foul, and we avoid them. It makes survival sense to eat what our taste buds like.

So eating is a source of pleasure. And what's more, it's now a source of ready pleasure. For human beings in the modern developed world, there's plenty of food about – such as the tempting, rustling packets on gaudy display in even the smallest shop – and we can have something to eat in our hands in moments. What easier thing to do than to eat when we feel bored or dissatisfied or annoyed or blue? After all, we are bombarded every day with minor stresses and irritations – travelling cooped up in trains and buses, waiting in long traffic jams, looking for a parking place, being shouted at by irate customers, coping with a grizzly baby, sitting at a desk doing a stultifying task. That little knot in the stomach might be suppressed with a few biscuits and a doughnut. Opening a bag of crisps will provide a distraction. Eating is guaranteed to make us feel better. For a while at least.

A moment on the lips, a lifetime on the hips ... Well, maybe just this one bag of crisps and then I'll stop ... And so sometimes we bargain with ourselves, make little deals. This slice of cake today then nothing for the next two days. Then the unexpected tightness of a pair of jeans we haven't worn for a while causes a stab of anxiety, a bad feeling in the stomach, which has us longing for a comforting bite to eat – but this, we think, is exactly what we mustn't do. We decide we need to lose weight, which means we need to get hungry. Hunger pangs become a positive feeling. Food becomes the enemy – standing between us and a perfect body. Our denial will pay off. We are in control and we will soon be a new person.

We'll soon be back in those jeans; we might even need a smaller pair. For a small number of people, this can spiral on downwards into serious, self-destructive behaviour, for which professional help is needed. For most of us, it's just another daily struggle.

Or we buy a bigger pair of jeans, or a pair of trousers with a softer, more giving fabric and a stretchy waistband. We've had a rotten day and we deserve our moment of peace and quiet on the couch with a snack or a drink and the TV on. We bought a 'value' pack but we don't need to eat it all at once. Hey, this is good – eating seems to be dispelling those undefined sensations of irritation, boredom and stress that were niggling in the stomach. We go into a bit of a trance. We don't even register any feeling of fullness because we've stopped thinking about what we're doing. We only remember what we were doing when we find that the pack is empty.

For a small number of people this behaviour, too, spirals out of control, and medical intervention becomes necessary. For most of us, however, our **bad food habits** have been accumulated in a busy life when we don't have enough time to think deeply about what we are doing and why, and **the good news is** that these habits can be changed.

Diet drinks
I have noticed that it only seems to be overweight people who drink 'diet' soft drinks containing artificial sweeteners. This is what I believe happens when you drink a 'diet' beverage: the sweet taste in your mouth gears the digestive system up for the sugar load about to enter your stomach and then your bloodstream. Your metabolic processes get the signal to switch from breaking down your fat and carbohydrate reserves and turn to the easy sugar hit that's on its way. However, artificially sweetened drinks don't contain any actual sugar, and therefore don't provide the energy that sugar would supply. The diet drink doesn't give you the energy your body was expecting. So after a can of diet cola, the sense of not being satisfied makes you more likely than ever to go off and eat some unsuitable junk.

Cave-dwellers in the
modern world

There is no question that we are better off than our ancestors ever were. Our exponential advances in technology, medicine and farming techniques mean we are comfortable and largely free from want. The long-term effects of this soft and trouble-free life are mostly beneficial, or at least harmless, but some of what we now take for granted is a mixed blessing.

We are surrounded by a huge variety of foods, but the easy accessibility of manufactured food, and the low price tag it often carries, means many of us are getting into the habit of reaching for the junk instead of the good stuff. This was not a hazard Stone Age man faced. But the price of not being killed by a lion on a hunting trip aged 10 or 20 may be a weight problem at age 30 or a heart attack aged 60 or 70.

Stone Age man was adapted to seek out the sweetest fruits available: sweetness meant ripeness, high-energy value and less likelihood of indigestibility. This adaptation is still with us today and is a fine example of how protective mechanisms can have a price. In our modern world full of sweets and cakes – chocolate brownies are my favourite – many of us might choose these over a piece of fruit, but the cakes are far sweeter than anything that would have been around in the Stone Age. Amid plenty, we are still driven by these early adaptive instincts. Fat, sugar and salt were all in short supply for most of our evolutionary history and people then would have been better off with more, rather than less. Where once we had to seek out – at high energy cost – what we needed, now it's everywhere. Foods high in fat, sugar and salt are not bad in moderation, only bad in excess, but excess is all around us.

But our bodies are remarkable things. Just as we are designed to eat, we are also designed not to overeat excessively. When we eat in response to hunger – real hunger, not emotional hunger – we reach a point where we feel satisfied: that lovely moment when you lean back in your chair and enjoy the delicious feeling of satiety. (Incidentally, a feeling you are more likely to tune into and relish when you are calmly sitting down to eat than when you are eating on the run and in a hurry.) Steady, continual overeating of bad food is not really what our bodies are driving us to do.

Eating the
wrong foods

A great deal of what we eat has been manufactured by processes we know little about, in factories we know little about, using raw ingredients we cannot always identify. Food technologists have over the years introduced colourings, flavourings and preservatives into foods, to 'enhance' their taste and texture, improve their look or prolong their shelf life – and then sometimes, with great fanfare, such as flashes on food labels, taken them out again. Additives are, of course, not harmful by definition. A favourite additive, which has been used for hundreds of years, is sugar, and it's even found in savoury goods. For example, canned and bottled sauces with a creamy base will only store for long periods if they have a low pH, which makes them taste sour. So a dose of sugar is added to counteract the sourness.

When we rely on food technologists for most of the food we purchase, then we don't always know what we are eating. When we don't always know what we are putting in our mouths, we are losing touch with our own tastes. We are not developing our own personal food knowledge when most of what we eat has been manufactured by someone else.

Retailers say everything they do is in response to consumer demand. But is that true? Have we become lazy and conditioned to convenience, allowing food retailers to choose products that suit their delivery and storage schedules? Perhaps we should examine our shopping habits and instead of going to a supermarket once a week and piling a shopping trolley high with a week's worth of packaged foods, we should shop two or three times a week for produce such as fresh bread, leafy vegetables, even meat and fish, if we are lucky enough still to have a neighbourhood baker, butcher and fishmonger. Many of us are lucky enough, however, to have periodic farmers' markets. They are becoming increasingly popular and even in central London, where I live, there are many to choose from, selling gorgeous, fresh, additive-free natural produce.

Eating for the
wrong reasons

Are you really, truly hungry every time you open the fridge door or biscuit tin, or just bored? Do you eat to calm yourself down when you get uptight? Do you raid the fridge when your partner/child/parent yells at you? But here's the deal: no amount of eating will ever satisfy an emotional hunger.

I have a very simple technique I teach my patients who are in the habit of eating without thinking. It involves asking yourself two questions when you feel yourself gearing up for a trip to the fridge or snack cupboard or corner shop:

1: How am I feeling?
2: What do I need?

Are you really feeling hungry? Probably not: so why are you going to get food? Aren't you actually just sad, or tired, or bored, or worried? Therefore, what do you really need? Some company? Pick up the phone and call a friend – this will probably do more to appease the troublesome emotion you are feeling than the food you were heading for. Perhaps you need the satisfaction of finishing off a project you have started, or getting a dull task out of the way so that it no longer preys on your mind. Or maybe you need to get a new project going, or take the dog for a walk, or sit on a park bench and watch the world go by, or do some work in the garden. Put some music on. Run yourself a bath, fill it with your favourite scented oils and bubbles and soak in that with the door closed. Or have an early night.

If you can remember to ask these questions – put them on stickers on the fridge and food cupboard doors if you like – then you will soon come to realize how you are using food as an emotional crutch. Once you have recognized that, you can learn to stop doing it. Try it. It works. It will not happen overnight but you will get there, as countless others have done.

Remember: this is not about distracting yourself from the business of eating because you feel you should be eating less! This is about recognizing that some of the triggers that make you feel you want to eat are not about food at all, they are about many other needs: for company, for task-completion, for relaxation, to let off steam.

Ubiquitous stress is a particular problem, and a common trigger for overeating. Channel your stress into exercise! Go to classes if you don't think you have the motivation to do it on your own. Kick-boxing and line-dancing are great, high-energy fun, and some gyms now offer cheer-leading and pole-dancing classes too. I like to de-stress by working out. If I have had one of those days, an hour or so in the gym grumbling, grinding my teeth and taking out some aggression on the weights is cathartic. And, of course, I like the results.

Most important of all, I want to get you out of a bad relationship with food and into a good one. That's what I want to show you in this book.

Keep a diary

Keep a diary of everything you eat for a week. Everything. You'll find it amazingly instructive. If you like, keep a food and moods diary too, and record when you feel an urge to eat outside of mealtimes and what might have triggered it off. Record what you ate, when and how much. Describe how you felt before you ate, immediately afterwards, and a couple of hours later. If you like, rate how you felt on a scale of 1 to 5, where 1 is a mild feeling and 5 a powerful one. This is a good route to self-knowledge. Once you know your own bad habits — there they are on paper — you can work on changing them.

Good mood foods

Many healthy foods have a high satiety value, which means they leave you feeling satisfied for longer. Mind, the mental health charity, are interested in how food affects how we feel, and they have sponsored research into the effects of a well-balanced diet. They found that the foods that delivered the highest feelings of satisfaction and helped the most in promoting a good mood were the following: potatoes, fish, oats, oranges, apples, baked beans, avocados, wholemeal bread, popcorn (plain, not sugary), lentils and rice. (Not a diet cola or a burger among them!)

chapter three
what shape are you in?

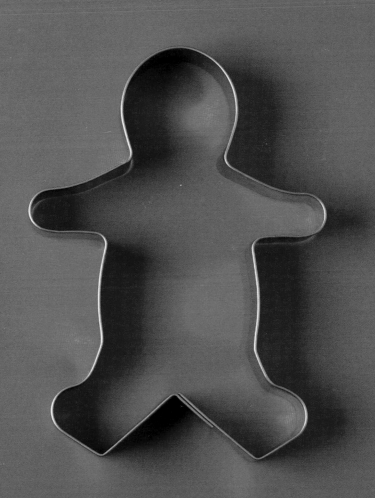

Do you feel good in your skin? **Or do you feel you are the wrong size when you go clothes shopping?** Is life so boring that all there is to do is chat on the mobile phone **or slump in front of the TV or Playstation? Is your main exercise going to the pub and playing darts or pool, or catching a bus to the movies to crunch your way through a tub of sweet popcorn?**

The shape we are in is determined by both who we are and what we do. We have hereditary features, and we develop habits. The easier the lifestyle we opt for in our youth, the more difficult life might be for us later on. Parents have a responsibility to their children to put them on the right path, and that doesn't mean giving in to them all the time.

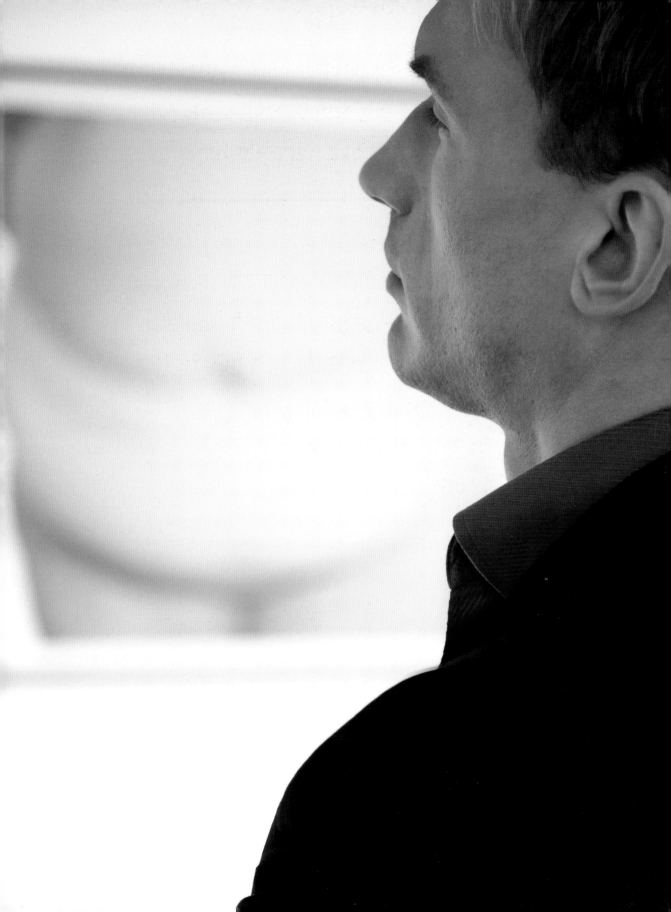

Issues with **food**

I feel that fussy eaters are not born that way. In the past children ate whatever food was on offer, just in smaller portions. Even today in many countries around the world children eat with their family, eating the same food as the adults at the same time. There is no choice, no special 'kiddies' meal and no attempt to disguise fresh vegetables. In fact, giving children a choice of special dishes seems to be a feature of the English-speaking world. Why ask a child what he or she wants to eat when they don't know enough to make an informed choice? We encourage faddy eaters that way. Of course they are only going to eat a restricted diet of white bread, chips, burgers and ice cream if they are never taught to try other foods. They soon learn that throwing a tantrum means they can have what they like. The best start in life you can give a child is a varied, healthy diet and a curious palate. Children who enjoy a wide diet of fresh vegetables, brown bread, rice, fish and well-cooked home meals stay with that pattern for ever. As adults they might eat the occasional 'unhealthy food' but in a quantity that is harmless and without any corresponding sense of failure.

If we carry on doing nothing about our diet it will be a one-way ticket to constant health problems that are the result of being long-term overweight or underweight, never mind the inconvenience and discomfort of being that size. The discomfort of being vulnerably thin with protruding bones. The embarrassment of trying to squeeze an oversize bum into a tight seat, followed by the even greater embarrassment of needing help to get out of it again.

Our bodies come in many shapes and sizes and the human race is the richer for the variety. Every individual has his or her own perfect shape, and it doesn't necessarily conform to the fashion of the day. The medical professions have various ways of categorizing us, and it's quite useful to work out where you fit in. If you've lost a sense of what's right for you, this chapter is a good starting point for working out your ideal shape, weight and energy requirements.

Instead of snack/buffet pork pie (75g) **270 calories**
19.3g fat / 7.3g saturates / 1.2g salt

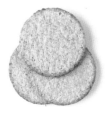

You could have 3 oatcakes **138 calories**
5.4g fat / 2.1g saturates / 0.06g salt

+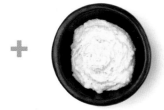

2 tbsp reduced-fat hummus **125 calories**
7.1g fat / 1.1g saturates / 1g salt

+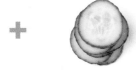

2-inch piece cucumber **3 calories**
0g fat / 0g saturates / 0g salt

total **266 calories**
12.5g fat /3.2g saturates / 1.06g salt

Calories = kcals throughout

BMI (Body Mass Index)

Your BMI is a measure of your overall weight, scaled according to your height. It's a simple formula worked out using metric measures (scales and tape measures come in both metric and old-fashioned feet and inches, stones, pounds and ounces, so for this exercise just memorize your particular metres and kilos). It's a useful, if approximate, way of seeing how overweight or underweight an individual is.

The equation is this: you take your weight in kilos and divide it by your height in metres squared. See the examples below.

Woman A:

A woman 1.62 metres tall weighs 63 kilos
To 'square' her height of 1.62, multiply it by itself: 1.62 x 1.62 = 2.62
Then divide the weight in kilos (63) by 2.62, which comes to 24
Her BMI is 24.
She is inside the good health range.

Man B:

A man 1.78 metres tall weighs 84 kilos
1.78 x 1.78 = 3.16
84 ÷ 3.16 = 26.6
The BMI is 26.6.
He is into the overweight range and ought to lose at least 7 kilos to bring him into the healthy range at around 24.6.

The BMI ranges

★ A healthy range is considered to be BMI 18.6 to 24.9
★ Underweight is anything below 18.6
★ Overweight is 25 – 29.9
★ Obese is 30 – 34.9
★ Morbidly obese is 35 and over

As with all set formulas, there are exceptions. Body-builders and thickset active sportsmen and women (such as rugby players) may have high BMIs, while marathon runners and ballet dancers may have low BMIs, but in both cases be fit and healthy because their body mass is lean muscle and not flabby fat.

I feel that BMI has its flaws, but for the average person it paints a useful and revealing picture.

supersizesuperskinny

Body shape Are you a pear, an apple or a thin chilli?

Medical experts have long recognized that as well as BMI there should be another category based on shape. The British Nutrition Foundation, British Diabetic Association and Medical Research Council recommend an overall body shape chart devised by Dr Margaret Ashwell, incorporating a waist-to-height ratio. Dr Ashwell's chart uses colours and the outline of fruits and chilli shapes for comparison. In fact, just looking at yourself naked in the mirror will give you a good clue. Whether your tendency is pear or apple, if you are at or near your ideal weight you will still be perfect.

Using your BMI with your waist measurement gives you a more accurate and clearer picture.

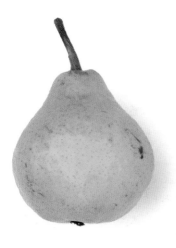

The pear:

many more women than men are in this category. Extra weight is carried on the hips and thighs. This is considered quite a healthy place to store fat, so long as not to excess, because it is away from vital internal organs.

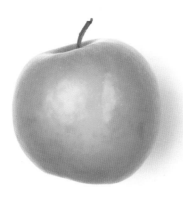

The apple:

most men and some women fall into this category. Excess weight is carried on the belly, waist, upper arms and breasts. This is a less healthy fat distribution because fat is being stored near to and around internal organs.

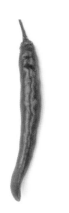

The chilli:

this straight up-and-down shape on a woman is likely to indicate that she is underweight.

Waist measures:
when you are at risk

Your waist measurement is another indicator of where fat is being distributed. Anyone carrying a lot of excess weight at their waist will be storing hidden fat around their internal organs. This table takes into account the common difference between European and African men and Asian men:

	Increased risk	High risk
European/African men	94cm (37 inches)	102cm (40 inches and beyond)
Asian men	90cm (36 inches)	
Women, all races	80cm (32 inches)	88cm (35 inches)

Body fat percentages

This is the approximate percentage of total body mass that is made up of fat, and can be measured on special digital scales. You can buy the scales for yourself, but better still, go to a gym and get an instructor to take a measure for you.

	Healthy	Overweight	Obese
Women 20–39 years old	21 per cent	33 per cent	39 per cent
Women 40–59	23 per cent	34 per cent	40 per cent
Women 60–79	24 per cent	36 per cent	42 per cent
Men 20–39	8 per cent	20 per cent	25 per cent
Men 40–59	11 per cent	22 per cent	28 per cent
Men 60–79	13 per cent	25 per cent	30 per cent

So what are the
healthy ranges?

For a woman
★ BMI 18–24.9
★ Waist up to 80cm (32 inches)
★ Body-fat ratio 21–24 per cent, depending on age

For a man
★ BMI 18–24.9
★ Waist up to 94cm (37 inches) or Asian 90cm (36 inches)
★ Body-fat ratio 8–13 per cent, depending on age

An expanding waistline might mean deteriorating health.

Your **metabolism**

We all need energy (calories) from food to stay alive – to breathe in and out, pump blood, think, blink and even sleep. This energy use at complete rest is your basal metabolism and accounts for about 45–70 per cent of your calorie requirements. Just as a car idling at traffic lights uses up petrol, we expend energy even if we seem to be doing nothing. (For more on metabolism, see page 86.)

On top of this is the energy we need to ingest and digest food, and the energy we need to move: to get out of bed each morning, get dressed, sit, stand, climb stairs and walk from A to B. Even the most indolent and pampered of us need energy. We need it to generate body heat, although in these days of central heating we need less than our grandparents did.

We also need energy to think and reason, because evolution has brilliantly moulded our superior brains. Every action we do requires some energy input. The more active we are, the more energy we need.

So our total energy needs are the sum of our basal metabolic rate (BMR) plus our active needs, including that used to process the food we eat. Anything we consume in excess of our needs will be energy left over. Extra energy gained from our diet is stored up in our bodies, some initially as simple sugars (glycogen) in our muscles and liver, ready for immediate use if we suddenly become active. The rest is stored as fat.

If we eat more calories than we need or use, we gain weight. If we use more than we eat, we lose weight. If we continue to lose weight, our bodies start to extract energy from our muscles by breaking them down. Then we become dangerously skinny.

Lifestyle and career choices also dictate our energy needs. Those who lead sedentary lives sitting at desks during the working day need less energy that those who do hard physical labour. But even the sedentary may need to factor in a burst of high physical energy during their leisure time either from jogging to work, working out at the gym in their lunch break or running mini marathons at the weekend. They may also lead active social lives, dancing, climbing, potholing, cycling, or juggling the twin demands of career and parenthood.

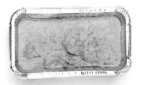
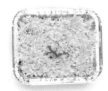

Instead of chicken korma and pilau rice (500g) 800 calories

44.5g fat / 20g saturates / 2.5g salt

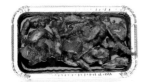
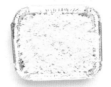

You could have chicken jalfrezi and steamed rice (400g) 526 calories

13.6g fat / 2.1g saturates / 1g salt

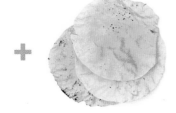

+

3 poppadoms 96 calories

0.2g fat / 0.15g saturates / 2.1g salt

+

mango chutney (1 tbsp) 80 calories

0g fat / 0g saturates / 1.3g salt

total 702 calories

13.8g fat / 2.25g saturates / 4.4g salt

Calories = kcals throughout

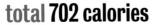

Our energy needs

We control our own energy levels. If we take in more energy than we use, by eating more than we need, that excess energy has to be stored somewhere – most visibly on hips, midriffs, thighs and chins. (As well as around our internal organs.)

If we take in less than we need to keep going, then our bodies mobilize energy from our reserves, which means our body fat and our muscles. This is why in extreme cases of near starvation, our muscles waste away: we literally consume ourselves.

The new diets that come out every year promising perfect weight control are confusing enough to send you straight to the biscuit jar. There are a bewildering number of rules to remember and most of them are tricky to fit into a family routine, or indeed any kind of normal life. It makes much more sense to have a good outline knowledge of what your energy requirements are, what your daily food groups should be and approximately what portion sizes you need, rather than worry about totting up calories or calculating points.

Average daily requirements

As a rule of thumb, an average woman needs 2,000 kilocalories a day, and an average man 2,500. (We tend to use the shorter form, 'calories', in everyday speech, though 'kilocalories' is the official term.) On this calorie intake, an average person's weight will not fluctuate dramatically – of course, everyone's weight fluctuates a little over the course of time. However – to press home the point – someone who has gained a lot of weight over a long period of time has steadily eaten above their basic requirements; likewise someone who is losing weight is steadily eating below their requirements.

The maths

There are formulae by which the specific requirements for people according to gender and age are worked out. Here's an example for a woman between 18 and 29. To establish her basal metabolic rate, multiply her weight in kilos (let's say she weighs 65kg) by 14.8, then add on 487. To allow for her physical activity during the course of a day, multiply this figure by 1.45. The result is her daily calorie requirement.

65 x 14.8 = 962
962 + 487 = 1449
1449 x 1.45 = 2,101.05 calories

If you have been seriously overeating or undereating, and you are aiming for permanent weight loss or gain, you need to make small, long-term changes to your eating habits. To lose weight, you need to reduce your excessive intake by 500–1,000 calories a day; this should result in a slow, steady weight loss of about 1 kilo a week. To gain weight, you need to increase your intake by 500 calories a day; this should result in a slow, steady weight gain of about 0.5 kilos a week.

Now put your calculators away!

Now that you are armed with the basic mathematical facts, and you know how the equation works, I recommend you put the calculator away and do not obsess about calorie counts. Think instead in terms of food groups and rough portion sizes, following the guidelines in chapter 7. Rely on common sense, and gradually tune in to what your body is telling you it needs. The more you educate yourself and your taste buds and appetite, the easier and more automatic it becomes.

Your body is a very clever machine, after all.

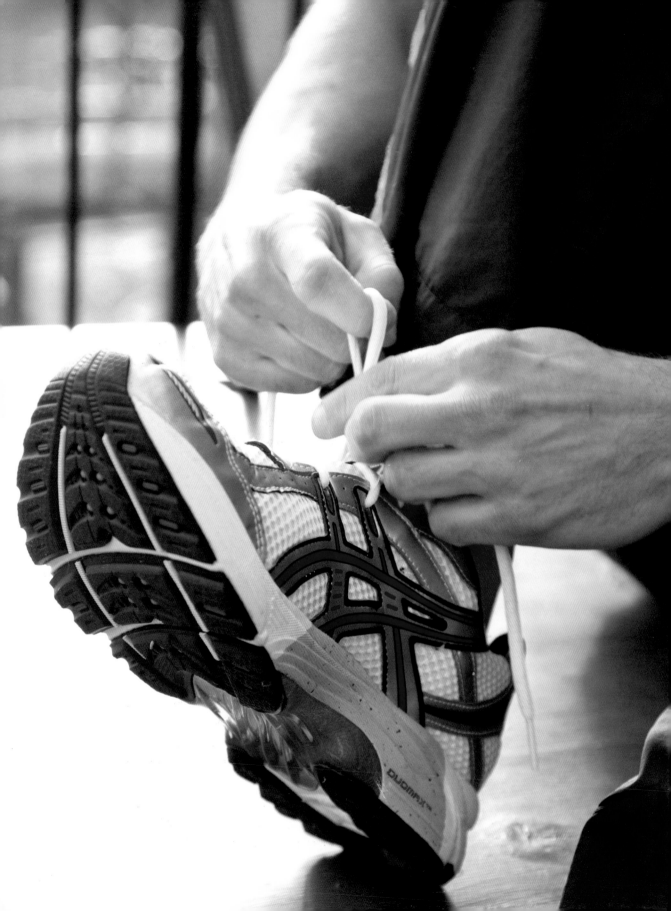

Exercise –
feel better for free

Exercising within your capabilities is one of the best things you can do. It releases powerful good-mood chemicals in the brain. It makes you feel and look better. Done well, after a period of time exercise will make you feel and look great. Your body gets toned and tighter and clothes start feeling more comfortable and looser on the waist and bottom. Exercise is a critical part of the energy equation. When we get food input and energy output in healthy balance, we maintain a steady body weight.

Exercise not only uses up any excess calories, it also has the added benefit of improving heart rate and muscle tone. It's a win–win situation. But we do need to feel motivated for it to succeed. And if you are overweight or obese and unaccustomed to exercise then you need your doctor's advice before you get started.

Cardiovascular exercises

The best form of exercise for weight loss is the type that gets your respiratory and circulatory systems working efficiently in tandem. This is called cardiovascular fitness or aerobic exercise. These are the rhythmical exercises – running, swimming, cycling, dance workouts and various kinds of keep fit classes – often done to music because that keeps the rhythm going. You feel a warm glow afterwards as endorphins are released into your bloodstream.

Walking is low-impact exercise, which means it's easier on joints. Start by adding short walking journeys into your daily routine when otherwise you might have used the car or a bus (or stayed on the couch). Once you've got into the mood, you can progress to longer walks, to walking for pleasure, even to power-walking during your lunch break.

You need nothing more than loose clothes worn in layers that you can remove and tie around your waist as you get warm: tracksuit bottoms and zip tops with baggy T-shirts underneath, a hat (to protect you from the sun or when it is nippy; you lose lots of heat from your uncovered head), a pair of gloves when it is cold, and of course a good pair of comfortable, stout, flat shoes. Many first-time walkers start out with just their everyday clothes.

Start off at your normal walking pace but swing your arms, gently at first if you feel conspicuous – though after a few days you probably won't care what anyone thinks, and anyway by this time you'll have started noticing how many other people are out there walking for the good of their health. Hold your head high and open out your chest. If you need to stop after a few minutes to catch your breath, do so, then start again. Give yourself breaks, and give yourself daily goals too: such as 10 minutes a day this week, 12 minutes a day next week, and so on.

It's worthwhile buying yourself a pedometer. They don't cost much. It's a small device you clip around your waist to measure the number of steps you take each day. Health experts suggest a good daily number is 8,000–10,000 steps. A 30-minute walk uses about 3,300 steps.

After a few days of gentle walking, start to increase your speed and the length of your stride and stretch out a little more. The best walking is a good long stride with your fists closed and your arms slightly bent, swinging alongside. It happens naturally as you build up speed, and helps tone your upper arms as well as your legs. If you want to increase the toning of your arms further, walk carrying weights of about 1kg in each hand.

Don't walk on an empty stomach. Eat a high-carbohydrate snack or bowl of cereal half an hour before you set off.

Running costs nothing except the price of a good pair of trainers with appropriate support (but it's not for the obese, whose joints are already bearing a great deal of weight). Buy trainers from a sports shop with experienced sales staff. Pounding the pavements can jar vital knee and ankle joints so protect them with the right shoes.

Swimming is one of the best all-round aerobic exercises with its steady rhythmic movements. It's good for the heart, for muscular strength and suppleness and, best of all, suspended in water there is little impact on your joints. To burn calories you have to swim at a moderate, not leisurely, pace. Start gently and build up. Allocate 30 minutes and take rests until you can build up to a full 30 minutes of swimming. The typical modern pool is 25 metres long. Swimming 40 lengths would mean you'd covered a kilometre, a good goal to aim for. For someone moderately fit, this can be done in 30 minutes.

Cycling is also good cardiovascular exercise but hazardous on crowded and potholed roads. If you wish to cycle purely in the interests of exercise, use a cycle track or the cycling machines in a gym.

Exercise classes come at all levels, from low to high impact, and are available everywhere from community halls to lavish sports centres. There are specialist disciplines, from yoga to dance to Pilates and to tai chi. Find one you love and you'll want to stick with it.

Racket and team sports – tennis, squash, badminton, football, cricket and netball – are good social sports. Being part of a team that relies on you is a great incentive to turn up.

Exercise is one thing that can dramatically change the way you feel about your weight, your body image, your relationship with food and, ultimately, your relationship with yourself.

chapter four

eating too much, eating too little

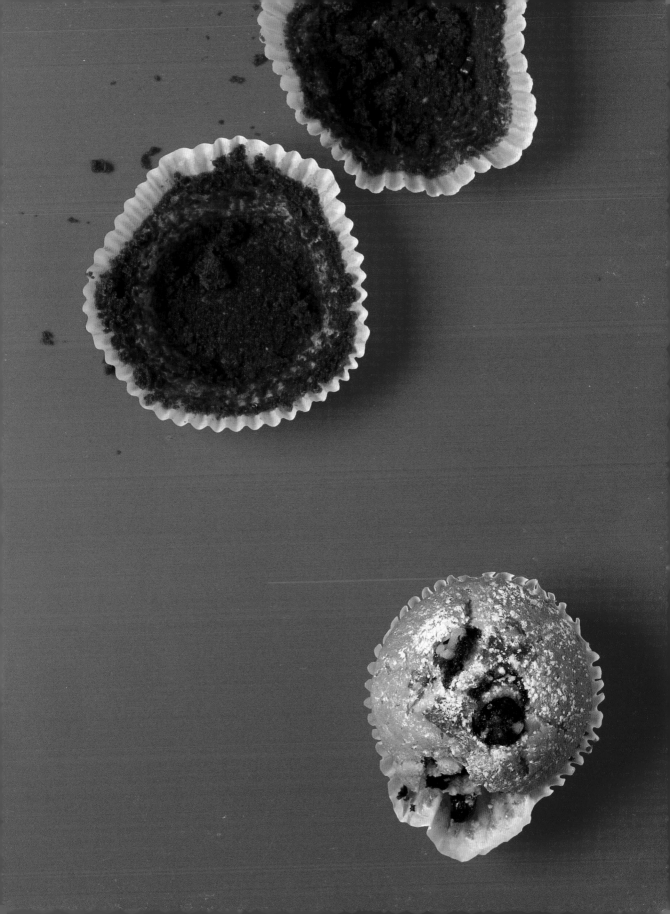

There can be no doubt that Supersize and Superskinny are in the same camp. **They may appear to be opposites, but when it comes to eating, they are making similar mistakes.** Both the underweight and the overweight I met while making the television programme were doing the same thing: depriving themselves of vital food groups. Neither of them was eating enough healthy food. Superskinny wasn't eating enough at all. **Supersize was eating too much, often junk food, and sometimes in binges interspersed with guilt-ridden periods of self-imposed starvation.**

One way or another, Supersize and *Superskinny* were allowing food to dominate their lives, and at the expense of their health. They were taking different routes but both lead to the same place: damage not just to their external appearance but to their internal organs as well.

Can we **see ourselves** as others see us?

Often, how we see ourselves and how others see us are not the same. The pressures generated by society can be so great that we start to develop a deluded self-image. There is an interesting condition called body dysmorphic syndrome, which means that what you see in the mirror is not how you really look. A woman who is underweight still sees her body as fat and carries on the work of starving herself even more. A man who works out and takes steroids looks in the mirror and still sees a puny guy, so he works out more and takes more steroids, eventually doing serious damage to his body. I suspect that there is a degree of this condition in all of us. Think back to when you were a teenager – remember when you got a spot and you looked in the mirror and thought it was the biggest thing you ever saw and that everyone was staring at it? We now know the reality was very different and in fact most people never even noticed it. But our perception at the time was quite different.

Working on the television programme which this book accompanies, I have seen the issues of weight and weight perception from many angles. For example, all the participants who wanted to increase their weight said it was because they were getting comments about their size from their workmates or friends and most of them hated being described as 'skinny'. They complained that outsiders seemed to have no reservations about telling them they were too thin, often in a semi-envious way, while they said they wouldn't dream of telling an overweight person they were 'too fat'.

The Supersizers disagreed. They said that people did comment on their size. However, they also felt it was fine to tell Superskinnies that they were 'obsessed' with calories and not eating carbs and that they were forever standing on the scales or picking at their food.

Interestingly, each side felt they ate a better diet than the other.

So we have a conundrum. Both sides insist they want to do something about their weight issues, and yet neither has managed to do it for themselves. Why? Is it that the pressures to stay thin subconsciously keep the underweight people undereating? Is it a lack of self-esteem that makes the overweight people not bother to improve their diet – they feel they are simply not worth it? How do we resolve these issues?

Plastic bags

Our stomachs are highly plastic, which means they can shrink and expand according to how much food we consume. In times of famine when our food intake goes right down, sometimes to almost nothing, this helps ensure our survival. Then, when the seasons change and we have food again, the stomach can increase in size once more.

And it is quite amazing how much a stomach can increase in size. Since we live in times of permanent feast, some people are discovering by just how much the stomach can expand.

Of course, we have regulatory systems to control how much we eat and to prevent us from overeating. Fat cells produce a hormone called leptin (derived from the Greek word for 'thin'), which plays a role in regulating metabolism and weight. Although circulating leptin is meant to reduce appetite, it doesn't seem to work with obese people, who can have unusually high concentrations of leptin in circulation without any apparent loss of appetite, as though they have developed a resistance to the anti-appetite signal. And indeed sustained concentrations of leptin from enlarged fat stores appear to result in the cells that respond to leptin becoming desensitized.

The effects of overeating don't appear instantly; it takes time for the excess calories to be stored as fat. So because we don't feel the effects immediately, we might think we've got away with it. But if we eat to excess day after day, we will gain weight. For every excess 3,000 calories we consume and don't use up in energy needs, it is estimated that we will slap on a kilo (just over 2lbs) in weight. That is the stark message. Regularly eating over and above our daily requirements means unused energy/ calories get converted into fat and go into storage, expanding our bodies in various directions: chin, belly, hips, bum, thighs, breasts, upper arms.

Compulsive eating

As we have seen, we often resort to eating to make us feel better and to keep us happy. One of the characteristics I have noticed in my patients who love food and have an ever-increasing weight problem is that they are outwardly happy and surround themselves with friends. Everyone loves them and finds them witty and great fun. But they know they are different from those around them and they have ways of deflecting comment. They join in the fun at the pub and make jokes about themselves before anyone else does. They wear big baggy T-shirts with 'I'm fat and happy' slogans and poke fun at any skinny people in their orbit or audience.

But the fact is that a compulsive eater does have an unnatural preoccupation with food. Very few clinically obese people are inwardly happy about their size. They know their health is at risk. Ultimately the solution is not just about making seismic cuts to their calorie intake. It's to do with their inner 'me' and how they truly want to see themselves. This takes more than just tackling their growing food intake. But those who find themselves in the compulsive-eating mould can and do make positive steps to climb back out of it, as our TV show demonstrates. What stars they are!

For most of them there is a trigger to take stock and change habits, just as there was a dim and distant trigger that set them off on this path in the first place. But they have to feel the trigger and want to make a change. No amount of nagging from anyone else will do it. This trigger often involves taking stock of their situation – such as watching their children growing up and wanting to be involved in their activities, like playing football.

Getting Help

If you are an extreme overeater, the first port of call should be your GP. You must accept that your eating pattern is not normal. Most GPs will be very helpful and sympathetic. They will be able to offer advice on self-help groups and therapy, as well as healthy diet. Or you can search the internet for self-help groups such as Overeaters Anonymous, who work on the 12-step programme.

You will be relieved to find you are not alone.

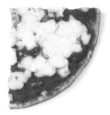

Instead of 1 medium slice restaurant marguerita pizza 270 calories

10.1g fat / 5.5g saturates / 1.4g salt

You could have 1 pitta bread 140 calories

0.7g fat / 0.1g saturates / 0.75g salt

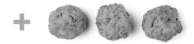

3 falafel bites 126 calories

9.5g fat / 0.8g saturates / 0.5g salt

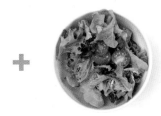

mixed salad 3 calories

0g fat / 0g saturates / 0g salt

total 269 calories

10.2g fat / 0.9g saturates / 1.25g salt

Calories = kcals throughout

mealswap

Superskinny's
myths

Our modern media world is obsessed with celebrities, who are photographed from every angle, any of which could be unflattering. The camera doesn't always tell the truth, but to minimize the risk of criticism, many celebrities opt for a very skinny silhouette. They follow a succession of fashionable diets and, frankly, crackpot nutritional theories, one of the more damaging of which recently has been the low-carbs message: that proteins are perfect because they build muscle (i.e. a lean food) and that 'carbs' make you bloated and big.

Myth: Carbs are just fattening. If I eat pasta I have to go for a run to work it off.

Starchy foods high in carbohydrates are a vital part of a healthy diet. Eating food in excess to your energy needs, whether that food is carbohydrate or not, is what makes you put on weight.

Myth: All carbs are junk food.

It is true that junk food is often high in (over-refined) carbohydrate; however, it will also be high in fat and salt, and it will have been so highly processed that the vitamin and mineral content is rock-bottom: these are the factors that qualify it as junk food. If I am able to show you nothing else at least let me show you this: starchy carbohydrates are good for you. Good quality carbohydrates should form at least half of your daily calorie intake: bread, potatoes, pasta, rice, oats, and so on. When you eat 'whole' versions of these foods: brown bread and brown rice, potatoes in their jackets, you are getting even higher levels of nutrients and fibre. Good levels of fibre help your digestive system to work efficiently, which helps prevent constipation.

Myth: Fats are bad for you.

Greasy junk foods are bad for you, that's true. Good fats, however, are vital (se page 91). We need EFAs (essential fatty acids) and good low-cholesterol fats to keep our hearts healthy. Every cell in our body is made of a membrane of fat. We all require a minimum amount of healthy fats for good health: up to 20g a day for women and 30g for men.

Consistent
undereating

If you look closely at the diet of a person with a very low BMI, it will frequently be one of lots of snacks or small portions of foods eaten on the run. A cereal bar here, a coffee there, some fruit an hour later, half a sandwich at lunchtime. All eaten in a rush, no time to sit down and enjoy a meal, even a light packed lunch. Eating little and often is not harmful in itself. It is a problem only when over the course of a day – and over the course of weeks and months and even years – it doesn't amount to enough food, if an adult is eating, say, the portions meant for a child. Not only is this person not getting enough calories, they are also not getting enough of anything else. Anaemia, for example, is a likely consequence, the result of not having enough iron in the diet. This can cause symptoms of tiredness and irritability.

Lack of calcium is another possibility, resulting often from a poor intake of products such as cheese, yogurt, milk and tofu. We must keep up our intake of calcium for our entire life. We need calcium for a great many functions in the body, including blood clotting and muscle contraction. If we don't eat it regularly in our diet our body goes to the next available source, namely our bones. Taking calcium supplements is not a good substitute for the real thing, calcium from fresh food.

Fibre is another possible shortfall – someone who isn't eating enough, or is on a low-carb diet, is likely to suffer from constipation. And if fat intakes are low, too, this can result in insufficient essential fatty acids.

Superskinny
bad habits

One of the bad habits I've observed in Superskinny people is that they will never clear their plate. No matter how tiny the portion they've taken in the first place, they will only eat half of it. Another bad habit is exercising too much and too hard, and not for the pleasure of it – because exercise can be a wonderfully stimulating thing – but for the pain of it, pushing themselves to compensate for eating.

A false perception common among the Superskinnies is that they suffer from food allergies and intolerances: sometimes one or two, sometimes the whole range. They'll claim to be lactose intolerant, or have wheat or gluten or nut or fish allergies. Of course, allergies and intolerances exist, and can be very troublesome for those who suffer from them. However, they are not at all common. They are very often, consciously or unconsciously, used as an excuse. It's a good one – who would argue with someone who says they have a medical condition? (Well, I might!)

More people are coming to me with what appear to be reactions to the pollutants in this modern world. It might be true that we are more sensitive than our parents and grandparents. But my experience has also been that some of these intolerances are more perceived than real. They are more likely to result from a simple dislike of a taste or texture of a food, which then gets extended so that an entire food group stands accused of causing problems.

My golden rules for
Superskinnies

1. Always eat breakfast

ideally high in carbohydrates (cereal or wholemeal toast) with some calcium, from milk or yogurt, fruit or juice. If this is not possible, then at least eat a quality cereal bar high in fruit and nuts and low in added sugar.

2. Try to include at least three healthy snacks a day

(see page 128 for ideas), when getting yourself back up to normal weight. Eat these in between your main meals.

3. Drink the recommended amount of liquid

1.5—2 litres a day, mostly water, but include tea and coffee. (In other words, don't keep guzzling water to stop yourself eating.)

4. Include good amounts of lean protein

at lunch and supper/dinner time as well as salads or vegetables plus carbohydrates like pasta or potatoes or rice.

5. Don't feel guilty about eating

enjoy the tastes, textures and colours of good food.

6. Keep exercising to within reasonable limits

and don't overdo the aerobic workouts and jogging sessions.

Anorexia **nervosa**

Anorexia nervosa is a psychiatric condition, with sufferers at the far end of the Superskinny range. Anorexics often say that what drives them to starve themselves is the sensation of control it gives them, while other aspects of their life, perhaps of their emotional life, feel out of control. Self-help groups and eating disorders charities are developing a wealth of advice and information to help sufferers and their families (see page 251 for contact details).

If you are concerned that someone close to you is in danger of becoming anorexic, here are some symptoms to look out for:

★ A significant weight loss for no apparent reason.
★ Never being relaxed around food: picking out pieces of salad that haven't been touched by dressing, for example.
★ Finding reasons not to eat with the rest of the family, skipping meals, or going without breakfast because they are 'not hungry'.
★ Being untruthful about how much they have eaten, if indeed they did eat anything.
★ In social situations, declining to take any food, even a crisp or carrot stick. (This is why normal eaters can sometimes feel uncomfortable around an anorexic; it makes them look greedy. Sadly this can isolate anorexics just at a time when they are suffering most from low self-esteem.)
★ Constantly worrying about their weight and size, weighing themselves at every opportunity.
★ When out clothes shopping, getting upset if they have to buy a size larger than they thought they were. And rejoicing when they can squeeze into a size smaller.
★ Drinking large amounts of water to fill them up, particularly before a meal.
★ Becoming forgetful or losing concentration.
★ Dependence on laxatives, slimming pills or diuretics.
★ Overdoing aerobic exercise, such as running, swimming, going to the gym for long periods at least once a day.
★ Spending too much money on clothes or trivial things. (This can make sufferers feel better for a short time.)

★ Physical changes to the body include lifeless skin that is easy to pinch into big folds, bony hands and feet, and the growth of excess body hair, especially on the arms as the body tries to keep warm to compensate for the loss of fat.

★ Some anorexics love to cook, bake and entertain but will not join in or eat what they have cooked.

Bulimia nervosa

This extreme form of weight control was recognized as a medical condition in 1979 and is now thought to be more common than anorexia. In the medical profession we classify it as rapid consumption of large amounts of food in one meal (bingeing), sometimes twice a day, followed often by vomiting. If it is not possible to vomit, the sufferer may consume large amounts of laxatives. Excessive exercising is common, as are violent mood swings.

Physically, the sufferer may start to develop bad teeth as the acid from vomiting will affect tooth enamel, and sores may appear on fingers through self-induced vomiting. The problem with purging is that vital nutrients will be lost as the body doesn't have time to absorb them and so it becomes weak and defenceless against infection. Continued abuse can eventually lead to liver, kidney and even heart failure. Sufferers may also self-harm.

Sufferers and their families should not delay in seeking medical help and counselling (see page 251 for useful contacts).

Size zero

Long-term starvation brings about extreme changes to the body. The World Health Organisation classifies anorexia at a BMI of 17.5 although most eating-disorder organizations would put this figure slightly higher at 18.5.

The international fashion industry is sensitive to the fact it is frequently criticized for using catwalk models with dangerously low BMIs, and some assurances have been made not to book models below 18.5. During the Madrid Fashion week of 2007, when an attempt was made not to use models with a very low BMI, the press went to town on the fact that around 30 per cent of models would fail the test.

The death of Brazilian model Ana Carolina Reston weighing only 40kg with a BMI of 13.5 brought the issue firmly into focus. The debate on using size zero (UK Size 4) models continues to rage. Banning models with an anorexic look may not solve the problem among sufferers immediately but it will remove a trigger that could help cut the number of new cases, stopping young girls becoming inspired by pictures of skeletal models.

I think most women would say that they do not like the size zero look and wouldn't want to promote it. And yet one large department store in London decided to try an experiment that seemed to contradict this. They set up a window display of size-10 female dummies wearing a range of different clothes. They kept the display up for two weeks and recorded the sales figures for those items of clothing. They then swapped the size-10 dummies for size-16 ones wearing the same clothes, and did the same thing. I am sure you can guess that the two weeks with the size-10 clothes saw significantly more sales that the weeks with the size-16 ones, even if the women were not actually buying size-10 clothes themselves – they just thought the clothes looked better on the size-10 dummies. But there is a twist – they also interviewed male and female shoppers about their thoughts on the clothes and the window displays. The women thought the size-10 displays looked best, but the men preferred the larger sizes.

Undereating is damaging to your health in both the short and long-term. Not only that, but it will cause the inner caveman in you to come out: altering your metabolism to protect you from this famine and ultimately making it easier for you to gain weight in the future. It will never be the right way to do things.

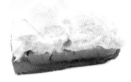

Instead of lemon meringue pie (95g) 240 calories

8g fat / 2.9g saturates / 27g sugar

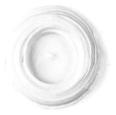

You could have meringue nest 54 calories

0g fat / 0g saturates / 13g sugar

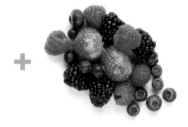

5 tbsp mixed berries 30 calories

0g fat / 0g saturates / 5g sugar*

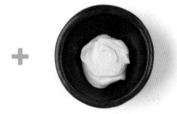

2 tbsp half-fat crème fraiche 130 calories

12g fat / 8g saturates / 2.3g sugar*

total 214 calories

12g fat / 8g saturates / 20.3g sugar

*Sugars mostly from natural sources (fruit or milk) / Calories = kcals throughout

Yasmin & Darryl

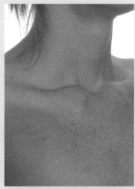

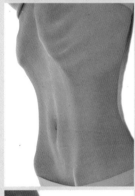

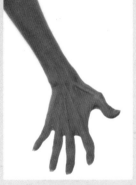

Yasmin

A 'too skinny model' who was struggling to find work because of her build, Yasmin had a BMI of 17.1 when she started on the programme, and was a size 4 on the bottom and size 6 on top. She weighed 49 kilos (7 stone 11 pounds), which she said resulted from her having intolerances to wheat, dairy, gluten and preservatives. She also thought she had an allergy to fish, and said that her whole family – her parents and young son – suffered from intolerances. As a consequence she cut out all wheat and dairy foods from her diet and said she hadn't eaten 'junk food' for a good two years, but did consume large amounts of fruit because she got so hungry.

Not surprisingly. When we analysed Yasmin's food diary before the show, we found she was habitually undereating by almost 700 calories a day. She wasn't getting enough minerals, especially calcium and iron, and she was also low on B vitamins, particularly folate and riboflavin (B2). She was eating too little fat and, because she was avoiding starchy foods, too little fibre.

On her first night in the diet-swap flat she felt quite ill; eating housemate Darryl's chicken dish almost made her cry. But she found Darryl 'great', really supportive, and by the end of the diet-swap Yasmin had learned a lot about her intolerances. She changed her daily diet to include more starchy foods, such as potatoes, and she cut down on fruit (to 2–3 pieces a day). One of her biggest changes has been to eat at more regular times, sitting down at the table with her son. She feels calmer, and is more relaxed and organized. She eats breakfast, and snacks on sesame-seed bars and nuts. Milk is still a problem for her but she has discovered soya milk lattes, which she adores and which supply the calcium she needs.

Yasmin is thrilled to have reached her goal weight of 54 kilos (8 ½ stone) and increased her BMI to 19.4. She doesn't feel as fragile as she used to. Now she has more energy to join her son in his sporting activities, walk the dog and play her passion – golf. She may even try to sneak her weight up to 9 stone.

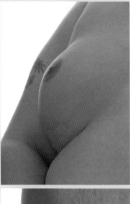

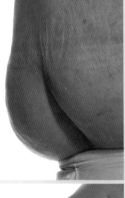

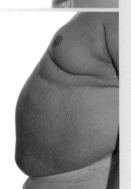

Darryl

Darryl called himself 'Happy Fatty' and confessed to being a compulsive eater. He reckons he has a good life – a job he enjoys and a loving family of wife and two young boys – but he was desperate to shed about half his body weight. Darryl is 1.92 metres tall (6 foot 3 inches) and at the start of the programme weighed 210 kilos (33 stone 1 pound) with a BMI of over 57. Bad eating habits had gradually taken over in his life, Darryl willingly confessed. He just ate and ate, and it was all the wrong things – mega breakfast fry-ups, 16 slices of pizza in one go, roast dinners with all the trimmings (including 12 roast potatoes), half a cheesecake meant for six, sometimes as many as ten packets of crisps at a time, all washed down with around six cans of diet cola a day.

The dietician analysed Darryl's food diary and saw that with an average daily intake of 5,300 calories he was getting more than double the amount he needed (based on the average of 2,500 a day for men). The volume of processed and junk food he ate meant his salt intake was four times higher than recommended (around 25g, instead of 6g) and his intake of saturated fat was worryingly high, too.

No one was more aware of the health implications of his diet than Darryl, and no one was more determined to succeed. The dietician suggested a gradually reducing diet plan, cutting down to 4,000 calories and then eventually down to 2,500. But Darryl wanted to go 'cold turkey', straight down to the 3,000 calories level, then down to 2,500. His first step – a big one for him – has been to include more fresh fruit and salad in his diet. He is controlling portion sizes carefully, and has almost cut the diet colas out for good: just two since he left the house and even then he didn't finish them. Now he drinks mostly water. No tea or coffee because he's never liked them.

What is making Darryl feel great is that he has been going to the local gym regularly and doing 15 minutes of cycling followed by 15 minutes of swimming at a good steady pace. He now enjoys swimming with his boys, and best of all he and his family have now enjoyed a day out at Alton Towers – at last, Darryl could fit into the seats on the rides.

His family have been marvellous, very supportive and encouraging. His mates at the pub don't tease him when he has a glass of water (he was never a beer drinker anyway) but he wishes they wouldn't eat kebabs in the car when he runs them home.

Andy & Amy-Jo

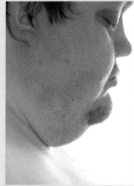

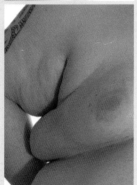

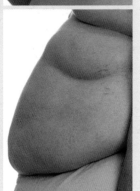

Andy

At 32 years old and around 244 kilos (38 stone 8 pounds), with a BMI of over 79, Andy said he never stood a chance of being anything other than obese because he came from an obese family. His 'before' food diary showed an average daily intake of 7,000 calories, almost three times the recommended intake. In 1991, at the age of 16, Andy was diagnosed with type-1 diabetes and needs four injections a day. At the time of his diagnosis he followed a healthy eating plan and lost around 57 kilos (9 stone) to reach 108 kilos (17 stone), but sixteen years later his weight had doubled and his health was in danger.

Andy is very aware of his size and highly motivated to do something about it, especially for the sake of his wife Anne Marie and four children, ranging from ten years old to one-year-old twins. Since his marriage to Anne Marie ten years ago, Andy has put on a stone a year. He tries to make light of his weight by offering to pose for photos for people who gawp at him, but in reality it is no fun and he is determined this programme will be a turning point. 'It has to be,' he says, 'nothing will stop me getting to my goal.'

His food diary showed that as well as a cooked breakfast, a big lunch and a substantial home-cooked evening meal, he also ate high-calorie snack-style food almost constantly. He drank sugar-free drinks and squashes all day, but very little alcohol.

His time on the diet swap was life-changing. For a start, he and Amy-Jo hit it off, learning from each other and staying in contact afterwards. And Andy realized just how far his diet had gone when he saw Amy-Jo struggling to eat his level of seven or eight big snacks a day. His daily crisps alone could add up to 2,500 calories.

The other food revelation for him was eating Amy-Jo's portions of fruit. Before, fruit hardly featured in his daily diet, and now he loves it. So when he and Anne Marie hit the supermarket they stroll right down the fruit aisle.

He now eats three meals a day and two snacks. The dietician offered to start him on a 5,000-calorie-a-day plan but, like Darryl, Andy found it better going straight to a lower daily intake of 3,000 calories. The regular eating plan he now follows is vital for his diabetes. And not only has he greatly improved his diet, he has also started making efforts to become fitter.

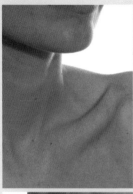

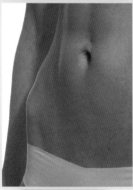

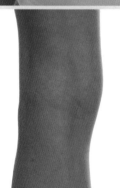

Amy-Jo

At the age of 18, Amy-Jo went into the event-organizing industry and started to eat 'rubbish foods' – eating on the go and grabbing what she could. After a couple of years her weight increased to about 57 kilos (9 stone), the heaviest she had ever been. Then she started eating more healthily and her weight came down to her current 48 kilos (7 stone 9 pounds). She's 1.7 metres tall (5 foot 7) and, at the time of starting the diet swap, a size 6 with a BMI of 16.8.

Amy-Jo's nickname at school was Twiggy, although she said she was never a fussy eater. Now as a 'yummy mummy', however, she felt her eating habits were becoming 'manic', especially her fear of carbohydrates. She began to diet after the birth of her daughter over four years ago and lost almost 9.5 kilos (1¼ stone), but thinks she's become too thin because she can see her ribs. Her goal is to increase her weight by 6.3 kilos (1 stone).

She also worried she was becoming a bit of a 'fitness freak'. Amy-Jo exercises for five to six hours a week in the gym, in addition to walking, running and indoor rock climbing – all of which require a high intake of energy from starchy carbohydrates, which she was not getting enough of. Her fire-fighter boyfriend would like a bit more flesh on her, she says, although he is happy she enjoys rock climbing with him.

Before she entered the diet-swap flat, Amy-Jo's daily calorie intake was 1,700, but her intensive exercise programme meant she should have been getting around 650 calories extra a day – in other words, she needed 2,350 calories, almost the same level as a man, just to keep her body at a stable weight. Although her actual diet was not too bad, she was running short of energy. She needed to increase her starchy carbs to maintain her high level of exercise and still achieve her weight-gain goal of one stone.

Now that she's finished the diet swap, Amy-Jo still follows the same exercise routine but with more starchy carbs to fuel her, such as a jacket potato at lunchtime, and toast with an egg at breakfast. She and her diet-swap partner Andy still talk on the phone every week, offering each other support and help.

Tracey & Alex

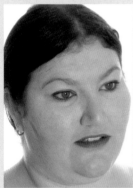

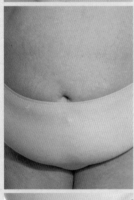

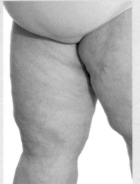

Tracey

Tracey describes herself as a fat Catherine Zeta Jones. She's funny and feisty, though she says she has developed this partly as a defence against comments about her size.

At 127 kilos (20 stone 2 pounds) and 1.6 metres (5 foot 4), she has a BMI of 48. She thinks her size might be the reason why she hasn't become pregnant, something she and husband Michael would very much like to happen. But Tracey finds herself surrounded by temptation both at home (Michael keeps spoiling her with treats like microwave popcorn, chocolates and sweets) and at work, a telesales call centre where office social life seems to revolve around the vending machine.

Tracey is a big eater. When she and her work mates go to a sandwich bar, they'll have a medium-size sub, while she'll opt for one double the size. At home she loves roast potatoes, frequently helping herself to treble-size portions. Between meals she snacks on all the wrong foods – kiddies' sweets like drumstick lollies, chocolates, crisps and all Michael's little treats.

Like the others in the show, Tracey found it hard to watch her diet-swap partner, Alex, eating her food. Especially watching him drink cups and cups of her beloved tea while she had to make do with water. And Alex's diet was hard for her to follow because it was based so much on sweets and chocolates with so little real food. She thinks she even put on weight during the show. One day she had to eat 20 KitKats for breakfast with a giant Galaxy bar for lunch. The most nutritious food she had was a bacon sandwich. It was tough, but she and Alex got on well.

This time, Tracey does not want to fail. She didn't like seeing pictures of herself in her underwear, and she's not looking forward to the show going out because her friends will see how big she really was.

Since leaving the diet-swap flat, Tracey has found it quite easy to eat the three healthy meals and two snacks of the eating plan, because it is very much the same food she ate before, just less of it. There have been some substitutions – instead of roast potatoes she has plain boiled new potatoes, and she packs herself a lunch instead of buying giant subs. As for her work mates, they have rallied around to give support, offering her grapes instead of sweets. Now she's just got to work on her husband to give up on the treats.

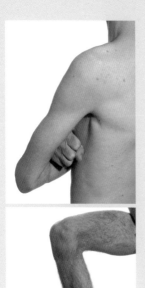

Alex

It was his mum who got Alex involved in the show. She saw how unhappy he was about being skinny, and he knows it is solely because his diet was rubbish. His height of 1.92 metres (6 foot 3 inches) and his weight of 63 kilos (10 stone) gave him a BMI of 17.6, well underweight. He is certainly thin, but not anorexic. He has no issues with food; it just doesn't interest him. But he does want to be more muscular and aims to put on a good 20 kilos (3 stone) because his job as a plasterer is strenuous, the equivalent of doing serious weightlifting and cardio workouts in the gym. He reckons his general health is not brilliant and it is hard to keep up with the physical demands of his work.

Alex lives on his own and doesn't cook for himself other than occasionally heat up a ready meal. He sees his parents about twice a month and his mum gives him a good feed. Weekends see him down at the pub, but he is not a heavy drinker, a few pints at the most, followed by a kebab on the way home. His mates give him some ribbing about his size.

Being on the show and seeing Tracey struggle with eating his food gave him a good outside view. He generally ate all Tracey's food, though the large portions were a bit of an effort, but he noticed that she did not usually finish his. At the end of his five-day stay in the diet-swap flat, Alex was delighted to find he had put on 4.5 kilos (10 pounds) eating Tracey's way.

After his diet-swap, Alex's biggest change has been in his shopping habits. Before he would pick up bits and pieces on the hoof, mostly unsuitable sweets and chocolates. Now he does a weekly shop with fruits, potatoes, bread, cheese and eggs, foods that need simple cooking. Before the show he wasn't a tea drinker, but drinking Tracey's tea gave him a taste for it, and now he has it at work. He eats fruit maybe twice a day, such as some grapes and an apple. He is beginning to enjoy eating muesli for breakfast. Before he would make himself a glass of a supplement drink or pop about three caffeine tablets on the mistaken assumption that this would help him release energy, but he had none to release. The big change Alex is looking forward to is feeling less lethargic. Regularizing his eating habits and eating three meals a day is a path he feels he can follow, and he's sure he will achieve his goal of putting on weight.

chapter five

why dieting is bad for you

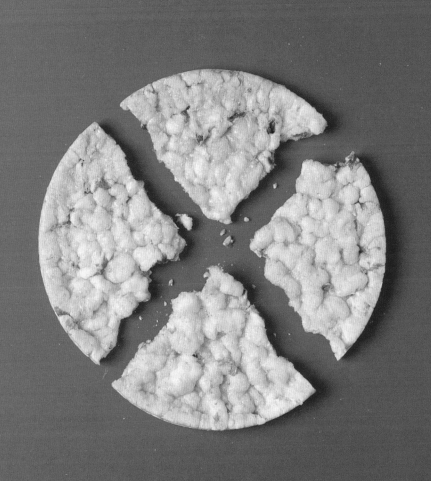

Your diet is what you eat over the course of a day, week, month, year. Your diet might be healthy or unhealthy, **or most likely a bit of both. Making your diet a predominantly healthy one is what this book is all about.** 'To diet' or 'to go on a diet' or 'to be dieting' is a process of controlling, restricting or artificially altering what you eat — often in an extreme or unsustainable way — in order to lose weight. **(Some people have to go on special diets to help them regulate a condition such as diabetes, but the vast majority of us don't need a special diet, just a healthy diet.)**

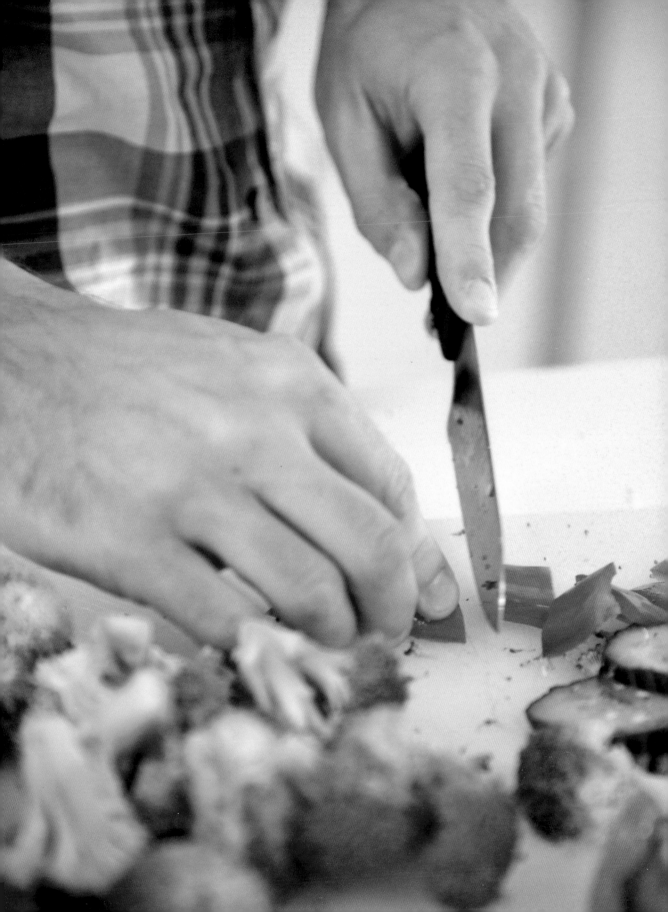

Losing **weight**

If you are overweight, then you need to lose that excess weight. You almost certainly want to lose that weight. What you need to do is learn how to follow a healthy, normal, gradually reducing eating plan that will slowly get the weight off and keep it off. If you are very overweight it's almost certainly because you've developed bad eating habits and, for you, changing your habits for life is the way forward. Slow and steady is the only way to do it. Exercise is involved too: not too much at first if you really are Supersize because your joints and your heart won't like it.

Around 90 per cent of people who lose weight through crash diets find it gradually creeps back on over the years, which is very dispiriting, not least because it means they subject themselves to the process all over again, and each time round it becomes even harder. Professor Kelly D. Brownell of Yale University coined the term 'yo-yo dieting' to describe the cycle of weight loss and gain. It's something familiar to serial dieters.

I'm not going to pull my punches here. Dieting will ruin your health and in the end it will only make you fatter. Right now, we're so confused by mad diets and bizarre ingredients that we've become scared of food. Sometimes we're even too afraid to eat the normal healthy stuff. There's only one way out of this mess and it's through knowledge.

A word about slimming groups: they can offer a valuable support system for people who need to lose weight, and some groups promote good eating habits for life even if they also endorse commercial diet foods. If you join a group, choose carefully.

Dieting will ruin your health and in the end it will only make you fatter.

Don't believe
what the dieting industry tells you

Crash diets don't work. They might provide a quick fix but in my experience they never work long-term. Your body has its own defences against extreme food deprivation. When the body senses that its energy source is falling away fast, rather than use up all its fat reserves, it starts using lean tissue and muscle. This lowers the body's metabolic rate, meaning it can get by with less energy, while it conserves some fat as a last resort. You need to work with your body, not against it.

And yet a lot of us are still falling for the false hopes and promises of the dieting industry. People are going on the wildest diets in an attempt to control their weight: many of them are expensive, most of them are potentially unhealthy in one way or another, and some are positively dangerous, especially certain slimming pills available on the internet.

We've probably all read about, or even followed, one wacky diet craze or another, when we were promised the earth if only we abandoned normal eating and drank a meal-replacement product instead. Diets developed to a formula are good business. They have been around for decades. They are sold in supermarkets and now online. You buy special products (usually at a high price) and plan your daily eating around packs of powders, cans of soup and sweet snack bars with added artificial vitamins and minerals. The newer ones might be more sophisticated than the older stuff, but it's an indictment of the shape we are in that there is still a market for such things.

These products stop you eating a balanced diet. You miss out on the benefits that fresh, natural foods provide, including important phytonutrients and fibre. And you miss out on the fun. You can't eat what your friends and family are eating; you have to eat your own peculiar stuff instead and probably endure a bit of teasing.

Slimming **pills**

Much has been made in the media over the past few years about miracle diet pills that claim to take the hard work out of losing weight by 'burning' up to 500 calories a day for you. In the States, slimming pills and wonder diets are big business, reportedly bringing in around $3 billion a year. All of these products use pictures of happy, slimmed-down clients and huge weight-loss claims to entice a growing number of desperate dieters. There are hundreds of these pills and products on the market, all vying for business, and many attacking each other on so-called independent diet review websites. Some have had to be withdrawn after intervention from the FDA (the Food and Drugs Administration).

An hour's exercise can burn up 500 calories and tone your muscles, improve your heart condition and give you a good burst of happy neurohormone endorphins — all for free.

Along with others in the medical profession in the UK, my opinion is these pills have a limited success and are simply not worth the money. Even worse, those who take anti-obesity drugs are often more likely to regain the lost weight later on. Medical researchers in the UK have warned against the sale of these drugs over the counter without a prescription because they are not convinced of their effectiveness. They feel it would encourage the situation that now exists in the States where huge profits are made without much evidence that the products are reducing levels of obesity long-term. Those making the products perpetuate the myth that popping a miracle pill will work. But it doesn't. The only things that work long-term are eating less/better and exercising more.

Don't even think of sending off for slimming pills that promise to suppress your appetite, 'burn' fat, increase your metabolism or offer any other apparent miracle unless you want to risk wasting a lot of money. It is believed that some appetite supressants can even become addictive. They can also leave you with a few other uncomfortable side effects like a dry mouth, an unpleasant taste in your mouth and dizzy spells.

If people lose weight while taking appetite suppressants, it is most likely because they are already restricting their calorie intake. And as ever, those with the largest amount of weight to lose, lose the most to begin with. It certainly helps the advertising claims.

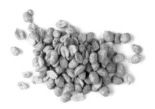

Instead of dry roasted peanuts (50g) 300 calories

25g fat / 4.5g saturates / 1g salt

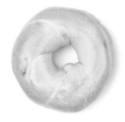

You could have plain bagel 190 calories

1.3g fat / 0.8g saturates / 0.9g salt

+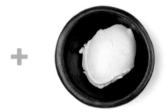

1 tbsp low-fat soft cheese 40 calories

2g fat / 1.3g saturates / 0.4g salt

+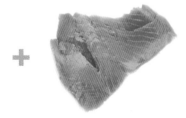

smoked salmon 70 calories

2.3g fat / 0.4g saturates / 2.4g salt

total 300 calories

5.6g fat / 2.5g saturates / 3.7g salt

Calories = kcals throughout

Themed diets

All diets work in the same way: a restricted calorie intake. Themed diets work by restricting what the dieter eats to an absurdly narrow range, which can reduce the nutritional value of the dieter's intake below what's healthy. The Cabbage Soup Diet, the Grapefruit Diet, the Apple Cider Diet, Food Combining, many variations on the theme of low-carb/high-protein – they've all come into and gone out of fashion. Followers often do lose weight, but potentially at the cost of their wellbeing, and if they return to eating normally they are likely eventually put the weight back on.

The main danger from long-term theme-based crash diets is malnutrition, which eventually damages the internal organs and bones. Take calcium, for example, an extremely important mineral in the body. We get it from fats and dairy products, in particular – exactly the sorts of food that are declared out of bounds by the themed crash diet. Calcium has various jobs to do in the body: keeping bones and teeth strong and healthy, helping blood to clot, keeping the brain and spinal cords functioning normally and helping muscles to contract. If we do not get enough from our food, our body starts to use the calcium stored in our bones and teeth, leaving them fragile.

Let's look at some of the themed diets. There have been hundreds in the past thirty years or so. In my view, many should carry health warnings.

Low-carb/high-protein

These have appeared in many guises over the past two decades – the Atkins Diet, the Scarsdale Diet, the Zone Diet etc. All were high-protein, low-carbohydrate plans promising – and often delivering – quick weight loss. The best known, the Atkins, promoted weight loss by a severe reduction of carbohydrates, and even omitted fruit in the early stages. Yet you could eat large amounts of animal protein. Digesting an unbalanced diet like this can put great strain on the body, especially the kidneys. The body is forced to get its energy from protein, a much less efficient fuel food than carbohydrate. These diets usually allow a high intake of fat, which raises cholesterol levels, and because of their high-red-meat and low-fibre content could increase the risk of bowel cancer.

The main risk of a prolonged high-protein diet is that the body can go into a state called ketosis. The body needs glucose, which is converted from carbohydrate, but if your body does not have enough glucose, because your diet has restricted or eliminated carbohydrate, it will begin producing ketones as it obtains energy from its stored fats. However, I do not recommend this form of extreme dieting. Ketosis can result in a strange smell of acetone on the breath and feelings of nausea. These high-protein diets do not suit overweight people with high blood pressure, kidney or heart disease. Also, as they are low in complex carbs, they provide an inadequate intake of fibre, leading to constipation and potential long-term harm to the colon. They could also increase the risk of developing gout, a form of arthritis.

No-fat Diets

Cutting out fats completely for more than a few days is not a good option. Your body needs the vitamins and essential fatty acids from fats to perform its normal functions. Women need certain healthy fats for their hormone balance, not to mention glossy hair and healthy skin. A very low-fat diet can leave a woman with fertility problems.

Food Combining (aka the Hay Diet)

This is not one of the worst diets. It was developed in the early twentieth century by an American doctor, Dr William Howard Hay, who suffered greatly from ill health. It's based on healthy foods, but on not eating certain ones together. The basis for his theory is that certain foods fight each other when combined in the stomach during digestion. The diet was popularized in the 1930s by an Englishwoman, Doris Grant, who found it beneficial for her arthritis (the one good side benefit was her recipe for a delicious wholemeal-flour healthy loaf, still in use today), but few doctors and nutritionists support the theory, mainly because once food is in the stomach, the acid used in digestion treats it all in the same way. People do lose weight on this diet because their calories are controlled but, with so many rules to remember, many people find it complicated in the long run. Dr Hay's health certainly did recover and he went on to live into his seventies but, being a doctor, he no doubt did minor adjustments along the way. His ardent followers didn't have his full knowledge.

chapter six

why eating well is good for you

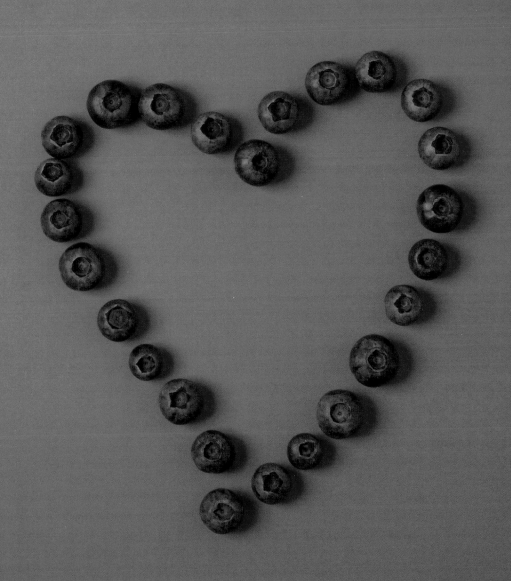

Every day, every single one of us, no matter our size, needs to eat. There's a hell of a lot of work going on inside our bodies just to keep us alive. **Even if you did nothing whatsoever all day – in itself, practically impossible – your body would still need at least 1,500 calories (for a woman) or 2,000 (for a man) just to keep ticking over.** You use up calories even in your sleep. **Eating is necessary and pleasurable. What could be better? All you need to know is what to eat. Knowledge really is power.**

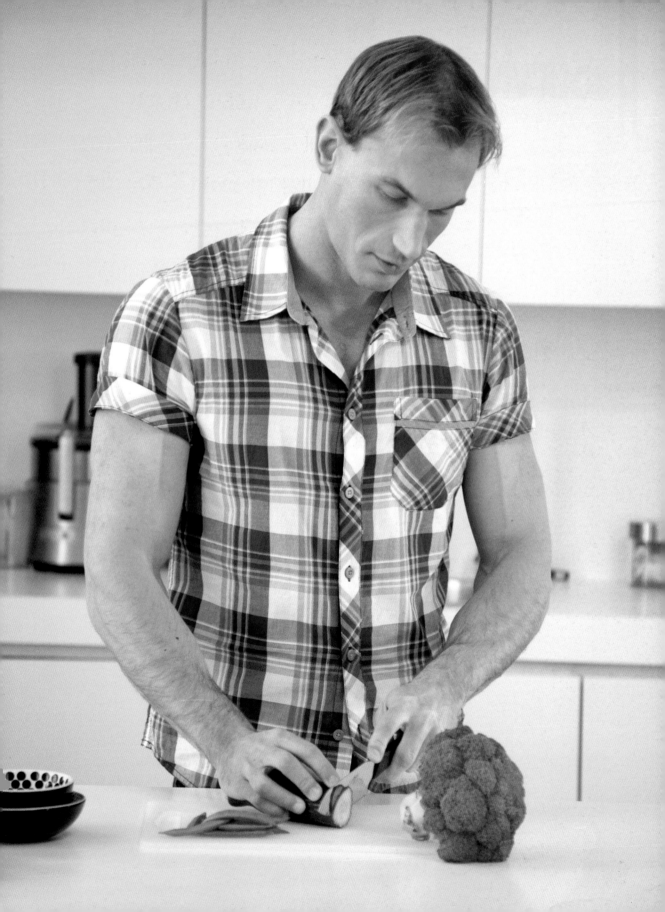

Survival

As our modern world of permanent plenty is relatively young, our bodies have not had time to evolve and take our new circumstances into account. We still have our prehistoric cravings for sugars, fats and salt, and we now need to overcome these primal urges and make our own adaptations to our eating environment. Each of us has to take responsibility for our own wellbeing. It may take a bit of time boning up on the nutritional basics, but they are easy to follow and you don't need a medical degree to understand them. This is your introduction; we'll go into more detail in the next chapter.

★ Eat three regular meals a day with a balance of the main food groups in each meal – carbohydrates, protein, dairy and fresh vegetables or fruits.
★ Eat modest portion sizes.
★ Always, always, always have breakfast. It doesn't have to be a full cooked breakfast, a bowl of cereal is fine.
★ Keep snacks, if necessary, to just twice a day and then small portions of healthy food. (See page 128.)
★ Eat a variety of colours and textures and flavours. Variety is the spice of life.
★ Make sure at least half your daily food intake is starchy (complex) carbohydrate, see page 89.
★ Eat at least 5 portions of fresh vegetables and fruit a day, not counting potatoes.
★ And remember to do moderate exercise for at least 30 minutes a day. Work within your own capabilities and limitations, and to begin with, go slow.

In this chapter I will discuss a bit of the technical stuff, in easy language, so you can understand what goes on inside you and understand what fuel you need and when. You wouldn't put anything other than petrol or diesel into your car fuel tank as otherwise it would splutter and grind to a halt. You should treat your own internal engine with the same respect.

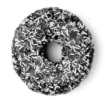

Instead of iced ring doughnut 287 calories

13g fat / 6.7g saturates / 23g sugar

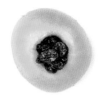

You could have baked apple stuffed with cinnamon-coated raisins 78 calories

0.1g fat / 0g saturates / 19g sugar*

fruit scone and jam 193 calories

6.4g fat / 1.1g saturates / 19.2g sugar

total 271 calories

6.5g fat / 1.1g saturates / 38.2g sugar

*Sugars naturally present / Calories = kcals throughout

Metabolism
and **calories**

Metabolism is often used to explain someone's weight: 'He can eat anything, he has a really fast metabolism.' We've done the sums already (in chapter 3), but how exactly does metabolism work?

I think of it as a collection of chemical reactions that take place in the body's cells to convert the fuel in the food we eat into the energy needed to power everything we do. Specific proteins in the body control these chemical reactions, and each chemical reaction is coordinated with other body functions.

After food is eaten, molecules in the digestive system called enzymes break proteins down into amino acids, fats into fatty acids, and carbohydrates into simple sugars (e.g., glucose). As well as sugar, amino acids and fatty acids can be used as energy sources by the body. These compounds are absorbed into the blood, which transports them to the cells. After they enter the cells, other enzymes act to speed up or regulate the chemical reactions involved in 'metabolizing' these compounds. During these processes, the energy from these compounds can be released for use by the body, or stored in body tissues, especially the liver, muscles and body fat.

Extreme dieting will slow your metabolism down so that when you do eat you will be more likely to store those calories as fat.

A balancing act

I see metabolism as a constant balancing act involving two kinds of activities that go on at the same time – the building up and breaking down of body tissues and energy stores. If you are undereating you will break down your body's energy stores to help fuel your daily activities, but if you are overeating you will build up those stores and lay them down as fat.

Several hormones are involved in controlling your metabolism. Thyroxine, a hormone produced and released by the thyroid gland (in your neck), plays a key role in determining the rate of metabolic processes in the body. Another organ, the pancreas, produces hormones that help decide whether your body's main metabolic activity at a particular time will be to build you up or break you down. For example, eating increases the level of glucose – the body's most important fuel – entering the blood. The pancreas senses this increased level of glucose and releases the hormone insulin, which allows your blood cells to use it.

The number of calories you burn in a day is affected by how much exercise you get, the amount of fat and muscle in your body, and your basal metabolic rate, or BMR (see page 38).

Blood-sugar levels

The term 'blood-sugar levels' is often bandied about in relation to the amount and type of food we eat. It's all a bit mythologized. This is the fact: our bodies keep our blood-sugar levels tightly controlled within narrow boundaries. Except for those who have diabetes or a glucose intolerance, these levels do not significantly fluctuate. Dizziness, headaches and irritability as a result of not eating (which we tend to put down to 'low blood sugar') can be explained in a number of different ways, according to the individual, but the answer is the same for all of us: sit down and eat something good in order to feel better! And see the GI information on page 106.

Facts about
metabolism

★ Overweight people frequently excuse their size by claiming a low metabolic rate. But the truth is it takes a high metabolism to stay big. The bigger and heavier you are, the more calories you need to stay the same size, and the higher your metabolic rate. When you lose weight by reducing your calorie intake, your metabolic rate slows down.

★ Our metabolic rate also depends on our age. Children and growing teenagers need calories to grow (even when they appear to be doing nothing except lounging around). But they should be growing into lean, active adults. If children and teenagers start to get plump they need to get more active and cut down on unhealthy empty carbs such as sugary foods and drinks.

★ After the age of 30, we don't need quite the input of energy we did as youngsters and we should keep an eye on our size. As we approach retirement age we need less energy still because we're winding down physically. We've raised families, done the hard graft at work and it's time to enjoy a well-earned break. Sadly though, at this stage in our lives our appetites probably remain the same, so we can go into an excess energy situation (this is especially true for women in their menopausal years). At this time it is a good idea to reduce portion sizes slightly and keep an eye on the scales, as well as starting an exercise routine or adding a couple more moderate sessions a week to compensate.

Eating a good breakfast will keep up your metabolism and help you burn more calories during the day.

Carbohydrates
and fibre

We all need carbohydrates throughout the day to keep energy levels up. To eat well, more than half our daily calories should come from carbohydrates, preferably complex ones. There are two types of carbohydrates – simple and complex.

Complex carbohydrates (aka starches) give a more long-lasting slow-release energy. They keep us going for longer. Complex carbohydrates also give us dietary fibre, which we need to help the body excrete food waste and keep the blood clear of bad cholesterol. We should aim to take in about 18g fibre a day, some of which can be provided by fruit and vegetables.

There are two types of fibre, both vital to health: soluble and insoluble.

Bran is a good example of **insoluble fibre**, which is light and bulky. Insoluble fibre is one of the most important foodstuffs we need because it keeps our guts operating efficiently. We also need to drink a lot of water to keep this insoluble fibre soft, otherwise we end up with constipation. The best sources of insoluble fibre are wheat, rice, oats and pulses. Lesser amounts can be found in maize, quinoa, fruits with skins and seeds.

Soluble fibre contains gums and pectin and once absorbed into the bloodstream acts like a gentle scourer, lowering bad cholesterol levels. It is a very important part of our diet. The best sources are found in oats and barley with lesser amounts in citrus fruits, pears and strawberries.

Simple carbohydrates, or simple sugars, appear in many foods and are often called the empty calories because they give us nothing but energy. They are the pure white granules (sucrose) we stir into tea or use in sweets, biscuits, cakes, ice-cream and sweet drinks. Brown sugars are still sucrose but also have trace nutrients in them such as iron, and naturally unrefined sugars can have a treacly flavour too. Simple sugars are also found in more nutritious food such as fruit (fructose) and milk (lactose).

The energy from all simple sugars is absorbed quickly in our gut and thence into our blood and when it is gone we feel tired and hungry again.

Simple sugars do not have a lot to do in the body apart from provide a ready source of energy, and if that energy is not used up by the basal metabolism or by exercise and activity, it gets easily stored as glycogen and fat. The more sugary foods we eat and don't use, the fatter we become.

You can spot the amount of simple sugars on food packs in the nutritional box. Here is an example from a cereal snack bar.

	Per 100g	Per bar
Carbohydrates	72.8g	18.2g
of which sugars	25.4g	6.4g
of which starch	47.4g	11.8g

Then set that against your Guideline Daily Allowance:

	Women	Men
Total carbohydrates	230g	300g
Sugars (simple)	90g	120g

Food is a gift we must respect and enjoy. It is vital to health, and eating a good, healthy diet is the only way to maintain a steady weight.

Fats

At 9 calories per gram (over twice the amount for carbs), fats are seen as the ultimate bad guy. But while fats are high in energy, they are also nutritionally valuable. We should never cut them out entirely. Our bodies need fats to function well. Fats also help food taste nice and give it a good mouth feel and 'satiety' value. We need fat to carry vital vitamins A and E around the body. Life would be impossible without any fats in our diets.

So we do need a certain amount, but not a lot: around 70g a day for women and 95g a day for men, and that includes the amount from all the foods we eat, not just what we spread on our morning toast.

Fats come in two main types – saturated and unsaturated fats (further divided into polyunsaturates and monounsaturates).

Saturated fats are mostly from animal sources: meat, butter, cheese, cream, etc. We call these hard fats because they are solid at room temperature. We should watch the intake of these saturates and keep to within certain daily limits – 20g for women and children and 30g for men.

Polyunsaturated or monounsaturated fats are found in vegetables and oily fish. They are the liquid oils made from seeds (olive, corn, sunflower), nuts (groundnut, walnut, hazelnut) and fish (salmon, herring, mackerel and the livers of cod, halibut). They can be turned into solids with the addition of hydrogen, a process known as hydrogenation (see Transfats, page 140). Poly- and monounsaturated fats are the fats that help protect us from heart disease, cancers and other kinds of ill-health.

Liquid oils contain varying amounts of Essential Fatty Acids (or EFAs). They are the 'good' fats that give us all sorts of antioxidant protection, help keep joints flexible and skin moist and supple. Without them we'd become creaky and wrinkled. EFAs are classified as omega 3 and 6. They help to reduce the risk of strokes and heart disease because of the way they act in the blood. They have also been found to help sufferers of depression. They are called 'essential' because we must get them from food; the body cannot manufacture them. The best sources of EFAs are oily fish (mackerel, herring, salmon, tuna and trout) and extracted fish oils. Vegetarians can get omega 3 from flax seed oil. Omega 3 oils work better with vitamin C, so the old-fashioned dosing of cod liver oil with orange juice was spot on. If you eat a good five portions of fruit and vegetables a day plus oily fish twice a week, you can forget about the tablets.

Proteins

Many of us think of proteins as the wonder nutrient and that if we eat large amounts of protein foods we will be in peak condition. We certainly need proteins for every cellular process in the body, but we only need so much each day. Anything eaten in excess of that is stored in our bodies as fat.

Proteins are often called the building blocks of nutrition and are made up of 20 compounds called amino acids. Eight or nine (scientific opinion varies) of these cannot be manufactured in the human body and so must be consumed in the diet – they are known as the essential amino acids. (The term 'essential' in this context, and that of fatty acids above, means that the body cannot manufacture the substance and has to get it from diet.) First-class protein foods such as meat, fish, eggs and cheese contain all the essential amino acids. No one vegetable (with the exception of soya beans) contains the full quota, but if you eat vegetables in combination with each other or with starchy carbohydrate foods you will get the full range. A well-balanced vegetarian diet with vegetable and dairy proteins plus carbohydrates will be just as complete in protein as a meat eater's.

Proteins	Guideline Daily Allowance
Women	45g
Men	55g
Children, 5–10 years old	24g

A portion of protein-rich food will not be solid protein, it will have other elements, such as fat, carbohydrate and water. The most concentrated source of animal protein is lean chicken, at around 42g protein for each 100g uncooked flesh. Beef is about 32g, salmon 21g, cheese 26g, and semi-skimmed milk around 4g per 100ml. Cream is a poor source of protein.

Compare that with vegetable protein foods. The highest source is soya beans at 18g per 100g cooked weight, chickpeas 14g, tofu 8g and pasta around 5g for each portion. Clearly you need a bigger variety of vegetable protein sources in a meal compared with meat, but this can come from dairy foods, grains and vegetables to make up the suggested daily amounts – and you get other nutrients such as carbohydrates and certain vitamins and minerals at the same time. We need to take in proteins daily.

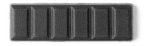

Instead of bar of milk chocolate (50g) **280 calories**
16.6g fat / 9.9g saturates / 29.3g sugar

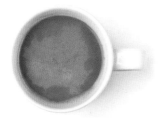

You could have skinny hot chocolate **130 calories**
1.3g fat / 0.9g saturates / 18.3g sugar

 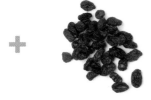

1 tbsp raisins 32 calories
0.05g fat / 0g saturates / 7.9g sugar*

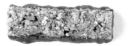

1 chocolate and nut muesli bar (23)g 100 calories
3.5g fat / 1.9g saturates / 5.6g sugar

total 262 calories
4.9g fat / 2.8g saturates / 31.8g sugar

*Sugars naturally present / Calories = kcals throughout

Vitamins:
a medicine chest

For the hundreds of functions the body carries out each day, it needs vitamins to act as catalysts. These vitamins also help to protect us from ill-health.

Vitamins are either water-soluble (C and B) or fat-soluble (A, D, E, K). Most water-soluble vitamins cannot be stored in the body in large amounts so we should take them in every day with food. The body can make some of these vitamins from substances found in other foods. The best example is vitamin A (retinol), stored in the liver of animals and good for eyesight, healthy skin and general growth. Not all of us eat liver, but if we eat orange or green vegetables containing beta carotene (carrots, peppers, sweet potatoes and mangoes, green leaf spinach and curly kale), we can make our own vitamin A.

The B vitamins are a group of six water-soluble vitamins used for our digestion, nerves and metabolism, among other things. Good sources are cereals, seaweed, yeast extract, lamb's liver, pork, pulses, oily fish and shellfish. They are referred to by numbers or names, and work singly or together.

Vitamin B1 (thiamine) releases energy from carbs and transports glucose to the brain and nerves. Drinking large amounts of tea or coffee can destroy this vitamin.

Vitamin B2 (riboflavin) also releases energy, from fat and protein. If riboflavin is in short supply then oxygen consumption goes down, which can impair athletic performance (which includes running for a bus).

Vitamin B3 (niacin) is another energy releaser, as well as useful for maintaining a healthy skin. It is one of the few vitamins that can be made in the body, provided you get the right proteins in your diet.

Vitamin B6 (pyridoxine) helps metabolize protein and, together with B3, works with the essential amino acid tryptophan to make an important brain chemical, serotonin.

Vitamin B12 – found in animal livers, seafoods and seaweed – is used to make blood and nerve cells. If we become very deficient in B12 we can develop pernicious anaemia. Strict vegetarians and vegans may need supplements.

Vitamin C (ascorbic acid) is the best-known vitamin. It helps keep our immune system healthy, and is important for building healthy bones. It is also thought to help reduce stress levels. A complete lack of vitamin C leads to scurvy (a dangerous disease suffered by sailors until it was found to be cured by doses of lime and lemon juice).

Vitamin D helps in the absorption of calcium for strong bones. It's found mostly in oily fish, eggs, some breakfast cereals and margarine. But we can make our own supply simply by being out in sunlight. Lack of vitamin D in extreme cases can lead to rickets (bandy legs) in children. Young factory children in Victorian Britain were the main sufferers because they were kept indoors and fed a poor diet.

Vitamin E is a powerful antioxidant and health-protector. It is found in nuts, especially almonds and hazelnuts, avocados, all vegetable oils and polyunsaturated margarines.

Vitamin K helps blood clot. It's found in green vegetables, but we can make our own in the intestines so we don't have to consume it. Babies are given a shot at birth in case they are deficient.

Folate (folic acid) is used in the making of healthy blood cells. Women hoping to start a family should build up good sources of this in their bodies before they get pregnant because it is vital to the development of a healthy baby. It occurs naturally in leafy green vegetables, yeast extract, breakfast cereals, nuts and liver, and it is now added to flour and bread.

Minerals make you **stronger**

We need small but vital amounts of minerals, 15 in all. Here are the most common, and the most useful.

Calcium is well known as necessary for good strong teeth and bones, as sufferers of osteoporosis are only too aware. But it has other functions. It helps muscles work smoothly and helps blood to clot if we cut ourselves, and a deficiency can result in cramps. We can absorb only 40 per cent of the calcium we take in, and we need vitamins C and D, magnesium and also EFAs in our diet for calcium to be effective. Dairy foods (milk, cheese, yogurts, etc.) are the best sources but there are also non-dairy sources: green leafy vegetables, seaweed, almonds, soya, Brazil nuts, chickpeas and sesame seeds.

Magnesium is a vital mineral that forms an integral part of over 300 enzymes in the body. It plays an important role in glucose metabolism, muscle contraction and energy production, and is also essential for metabolizing carbohydrates. A deficit of this mineral could leave you tired with poor appetite, weak muscles and an irregular heart beat. But if you live in a hard water area it's in the tap water so there is no need to spend vast fortunes on bottled water or supplements. Get it for free.

Iron carries oxygen in the blood. It helps wounds heal and keeps energy levels up. A lack of it leaves us in danger of becoming anaemic and unable to make haemoglobin. Women need good supplies of iron during their periods. It is widely available in many sources including red meats (especially liver and kidneys), green leafy vegetables, dried apricots, soya beans, seaweed, egg yolks, haricot beans, dried ginger and even curry powder. Enough to satisfy carnivores and vegetarians alike. Interestingly, calcium and tannin-containing drinks can reduce your ability to absorb iron, and this may explain why, in this nation of tea-drinkers, some older women are anaemic, even after their periods have stopped.

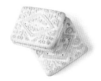

Instead of 2 custard cream biscuits **106 calories**

4.5g fat / 2.4g saturates / 7.4g sugar

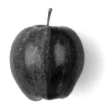

You could have apple **47 calories**

0.1g fat / 0g saturates / 11.2g sugar*

satsuma **25 calories**

0.1g fat / 0g saturates / 5.7g sugar*

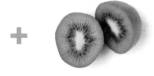

kiwi fruit **29 calories**

0.3g fat / 0g saturates / 5.9g sugar*

total **101 calories**

0.5g fat / 0g saturates / 22.8g sugar*

*Sugars naturally present / Calories = kcals throughout

mealswap

Selenium: a tiny amount of this gives us big health benefits. One of the important antioxidants, it helps protect us from heart disease, cancers and even premature ageing. It works in partnership with vitamin E and is found mainly in plants that grow in selenium-rich soils. Brazil nuts are the best-known source (ten times more than other sources or nuts). Others are mushrooms and the humble lentil.

Zinc plays a part in many of the body's functions. It is particularly important for reproductive health in both sexes, helps in healing and keeps skin fresh and healthy. It is an effective antioxidant too in the fight against free radicals (see below). Wheatgerm is the best source but this is not always easy to find, so look for it in meat and dairy foods. Pecan nuts, pulses, oysters and mussels, sesame and sunflower seeds contain usable amounts too. Boys who are deficient in zinc before puberty can experience delayed sexual development.

Potassium, sodium and chloride all work together for the normal functioning of cells and organs. They are important for maintaining fluid balance in the body, and are freely available in many foods. Potassium plays an important role in the functioning of nerves and muscles, including the heart. We don't need to take any trouble seeking out foods high in these minerals. But we should all keep our salt levels down to around a teaspoon a day (that includes processed and ready-made dishes). If you cut down on sodium for blood-pressure reasons, then eat bananas, dried fruits and pulses to keep potassium levels constant.

Antioxidants

When the body turns food into energy it produces unstable groups of atoms and molecules called free radicals, which can cause oxidation of molecules in your body and can, in excess, have harmful effects. Certain vitamins and minerals, known as antioxidants, can protect from an excess of free radicals by mopping them up so they can no longer cause any cell damage. If you can keep your levels of antioxidants high they will be able to neutralize the maverick free radicals before they can do any harm. See the Really Good Foods chart (overleaf) for good sources.

Trace elements and phytochemicals

Many of the nutrients we need to stay healthy are required in tiny quantities and are called, appropriately enough, trace elements or micronutrients. Some are antioxidants and so help in the prevention of cancers. There are thousands of them but here are a few of the more often-mentioned names: beta carotene (in many foods), lypocene (tomatoes), lutein, flavonoids, rutin, quercetin (in black tea), allicin (onions), isoflavones, capsaicin (chillies), anthocyanin (red cabbage, blueberries, cranberries).

The simplest and most effective way to ensure you get all these vital little nutrients is to eat a daily variety of fresh fruit and vegetables — at least five portions a day. Eat a good mixture in a varied diet and you can forget the science.

Really good foods

Food	Nutrients	What it does for You	Portion size
Almonds	Calcium, zinc, vit E	Good non-dairy source of calcium	10 nuts
Apples	Vit C, phytonutrient quercetin	Antioxidant for general wellbeing and helps protect against cancer and heart disease	1 med size
	Soluble fibre	Lowers blood cholesterol	
Apricots, dried	Beta carotene (which the body turns into vit A)	Helps protect against cancer and heart disease	50g dried
Asparagus	Asparagine, beta carotene	Natural diuretic and anti-inflammatory	100g / ⅓ bunch
Avocados	Vit E, potassium, monounsaturated fats	Helps protect against heart disease and lower blood cholesterol	½ med size
Bananas	Potassium	Regulates blood pressure. Good for the heart	1 small

Food	Nutrients	What it does for You	Portion size
Barley – pearl/pot	Vit B6, iron, insoluble fibre	Helps to lower blood cholesterol	50g dried
Blackberries	Vit E, antioxidants	Helps protect against cancer	100g fresh
Blackcurrants	Anthocyanins, vit C	Helps protect against cancer and heart disease, very high vit C	100g fresh
Blueberries	Vit C, manganese	Helps protect against cancer and heart disease	100g fresh
Brazil nuts	Selenium, zinc, magnesium	Selenium is a high rate antioxidant. Zinc is good for the natural immune system	50g shelled
Broad beans	Insoluble fibre, beta carotene, potassium	Helps reduce blood cholesterol especially if inner skins retained	100g fresh or frozen
Broccoli	Folate (for folic acid), beta carotene, antioxidants	Helps protect against cancer. Good in pregnancy	100g (half small head)
Brussels sprouts	Antioxidants, folate, beta carotene	Helps protect against cancer. Good in pregnancy	100g fresh or frozen
Butternut squash	Beta carotene	Protects against cancer and heart disease	100g (peeled and seeded)

Food	Nutrients	What it does for You	Portion size
Cabbage	Beta carotene, folate	Helps protect against cancer. Eat dark leaves for best source	100g fresh
Cashew nuts	Selenium, zinc, magnesium	See brazils	50g unsalted
Cherries	Anthocyanins	Natural antioxidants. Helps protect against cancer and heart disease	100g fresh
Chillies, fresh	Capsaicin	Anti-inflammatory, helps speed up metabolism and lower blood cholesterol	To taste
Cranberries	Antiviral properties, manganese	The saviour of those who suffer the misery of urinary tract infections	1 small glass unsweetened juice 50g dried berries
Flour, wholemeal	B group vits, fibre	Low GI if 100% wholemeal. Good source of fibre	50g
Garlic, fresh	Allicin, antiviral properties, antifungal, antioxidants	Helps protect against heart disease	1–2 fat cloves
Ginger root	Zingerone	Aids digestion, reduces travel sickness and morning sickness	2cm piece
Grapes, red	Anthocyanins	Antioxidant to protect against heart disease	small 50g bunch

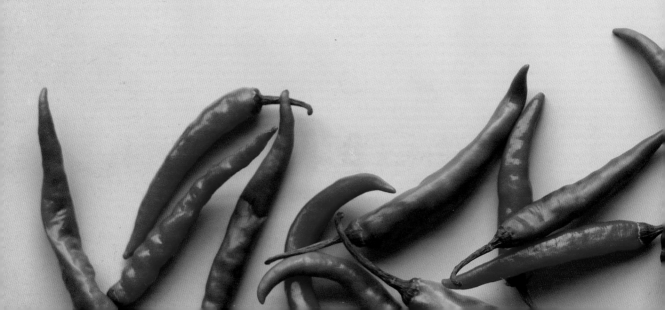

Food	Nutrients	What it does for You	Portion size
Grapefruit, pink	Beta carotene	Antioxidant to protect heart	½ fresh
Hazelnuts	Like cashews and brazils	Antioxidant to protect heart	50g
Honey	High in fructose (natural fruit sugar)	Antibacterial. Known in ancient days as the healer	2 tsp
Kale	Vits A, C, E	Natural antioxidants, esp. in dark leaves, helps protect against cancer	100g fresh
Kiwi fruit	Vit C	One of the best sources of vitamin C	1 medium fruit
Lentils	Insoluble fibre	Good, low-fat source protein, especially when eaten with starchy food. Maintains healthy digestive system	50g dry weight
Mangoes	Vit E, potassium, beta carotene	High in soluble fibre to help lower blood cholesterol. Good antioxidants	½ med size
Melon, red and orange only	Beta carotene, potassium	Good antioxidants	1 good slice
Mussels	Zinc, selenium, magnesium	Low-calorie protein, high in antioxidants and omega 3 (unlike other shellfish)	100g shelled
Oily fish: salmon, sardines, herring, mackerel	Omega 3 fatty acids	Helps protect heart; eat twice weekly	100g filleted

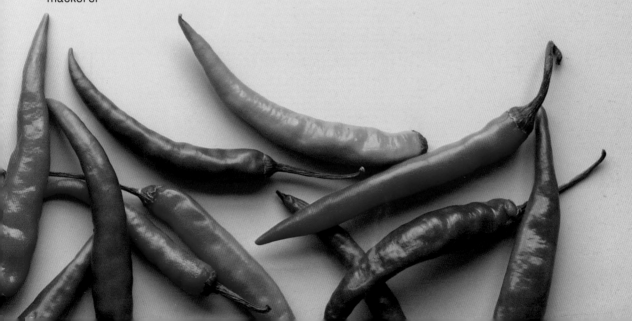

Food	Nutrients	What it does for You	Portion size
Oats	Soluble fibre, manganese	Helps to lower cholesterol in the blood. Good for a healthy heart	30g dry weight (3–4 tbsp)
Olive oil	Monounsaturated fatty acids	Helps to lower blood cholesterol levels and good for a healthy heart	1–2 tsp
Onions, inc. spring onions	Allicin	Helps to lower blood pressure and cholesterol and build resistance	½ med onion
Oranges	Vit C and antioxidants	Helps to prevent cancer. Also good for general wellbeing	1 med
Papaya	Beta carotene, vit C	Good in antioxidants to help prevent cancers and heart disease. Sometimes used as a fat replacement in baking	½ fresh
Pasta, wholewheat	Low GI, B group vits	Good for slow energy release and for dietary fibre for the digestive system	50g dry weight
Peas, fresh and frozen	Vit C, fibre, potassium, folate	For general good health, and good for digestive system	100g
Peppers, green	Vit C	Natural antioxidants to help protect against cancer	½ fresh
Peppers, red	Vit C and beta carotene		½ fresh
Quinoa grains	Calcium, iron	For healthy bones. Iron carries oxygen around the body. Good alternative to couscous and rice	50g dry weight
Raspberries	Many phytonutrients, vit C	Natural antioxidants to help protect against cancer	100g
Rice, brown basmati	Good source of dietary fibre, B group vits	Good for digestive system	50g dry weight
Seaweeds, e.g. nori/laverbread, kombu	Iodine, calcium, iron	Good for bones and teeth and for carrying oxygen around in the blood	1 tbsp dried

Food	Nutrients	What it does for You	Portion size
Seeds, sesame	Calcium	Good for healthy bones and teeth	1–2 tsp
Seeds, sunflower	Vit E, B group vits, iron, copper, polyunsaturated fats	Helps protect against heart disease	2 tsp
Soya and dried beans/pulses	Phytonutrients, antioxidants	Soya is a complete vegetable protein with all amino acids. Other beans are good sources of fibre for digestive system. Soya milk is low in fat and high in protein	100g cooked
Squash and sweet potatoes	All antioxidants, beta carotene, vits C and E	Helps protect against cancers and heart disease	100g peeled weight
Tea	Phytonutrients, fluoride	Helps protect against cancers and heart disease. Fluoride helps prevent tooth decay	No more than 5 cups a day
Tomatoes	Antioxidant, phytonutrient lycopene	Helps protects against cancer and heart disease. Stronger in cooked form	1 fresh or 1 tbsp ketchup
Walnuts	Vit E	Helps protect against heart disease	50g
Watercress	Antioxidants, vits B and C, iron	Helps protect against cancers and heart disease	½ bunch at least, more than a garnish

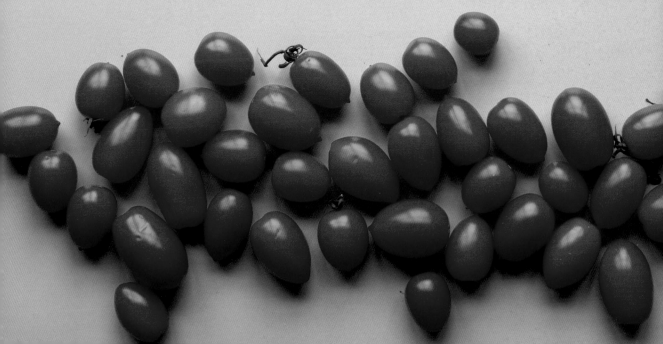

The GI diet

There is a diet tool that is gaining support among health professionals – the one that measures the Glycaemic Index (GI) of carbohydrate-containing foods. This is a ranking based on the rate at which carbohydrates raise blood-sugar levels. It has been developed to help diabetics manage their sugar levels during mealtimes but is now used as a good general guide to healthy balanced eating for us all.

All foods that contain carbohydrate are divided according to an index of low, medium or high. A food that is broken down quickly, releasing glucose rapidly into the bloodstream, will have a high GI level. Glucose (the carbohydrate that is absorbed the quickest) is set at a GI of 100.

Carbohydrates that are broken down slowly in digestion are given a low GI value. It is thought that slow, steady rises and falls in blood-sugar levels can help you feel full for longer and so help with weight management. For this reason low and medium GI foods are more satisfying than those with high GI. So it becomes quite an easy formula to remember.

The GI index of a meal may also be affected by the amount of fat or protein (meat, fish, eggs) eaten at the same time, which slows down the rate of absorption into the body, and by the type of sugar. Fructose (fruit sugar) and lactose (from milk) take longer to be absorbed than sucrose, and acidic fruits like lemon or orange juice also slow down the absorption rate. The way food is cooked or processed can also affect the GI.

Here is a useful list so you can plan your daily intake. But please don't exclude foods from the high GI category – just eat them in moderation in a combination with protein and fat foods.

High GI foods – eat occasionally, ideally with lean protein or low-fat food

High GI foods include over-refined foods made with white flour and sugar such as white bread, biscuits, sweets, cornflakes, white rice, rice cakes, crackers, doughnuts (no surprises there), Rice Krispies, watermelon, parsnips, microwaved baked potatoes, dates.

Medium GI foods – eat often

Medium GI foods are the pastas, brown rices, digestive biscuits, Ryvita, pitta breads, mangoes, pineapple, raisins, boiled potatoes, spaghetti, muesli, Shredded Wheat, basmati rice.

Low GI foods – favour these in your diet

Low GI foods are those that slowly release sugar into the blood. Often these foods also contain good amounts of dietary fibre. Eating low GI foods can help to keep your daily energy levels balanced. They include all pulses (including baked beans), certain fruits such as apples, plums and peaches, and most vegetables. Peanuts, soy beans, lentils, kidney beans, chickpeas, courgettes, tomatoes, vegetable squashes, peppers, lettuce, avocados, aubergines, green beans, cucumber, celery, cauliflower, broccoli, asparagus, canned tomato soup, cooked carrots, wholewheat pasta, bananas, dried apricots, kiwis, cherries, grapefruit, all dairy foods (inc low-fat, sugar-free yogurt), soya milk, pearl barley, porridge oats, All-Bran, wholemeal bread, multigrain bread, fruit juices.

There are some surprises, in particular cooked potatoes, because the cooking method can also influence the rate at which starchy carbohydrates are absorbed into the blood. Plain boiled potatoes have a medium GI rating because the starch takes some time to digest. But if you mash those boiled potatoes you alter the rate at which they are broken down and absorbed and so they assume a higher GI rating. As do baked potatoes. However, serving baked potatoes with a lower GI food like baked beans will lower the GI of the meal.

chapter seven

one eating plan for everyone

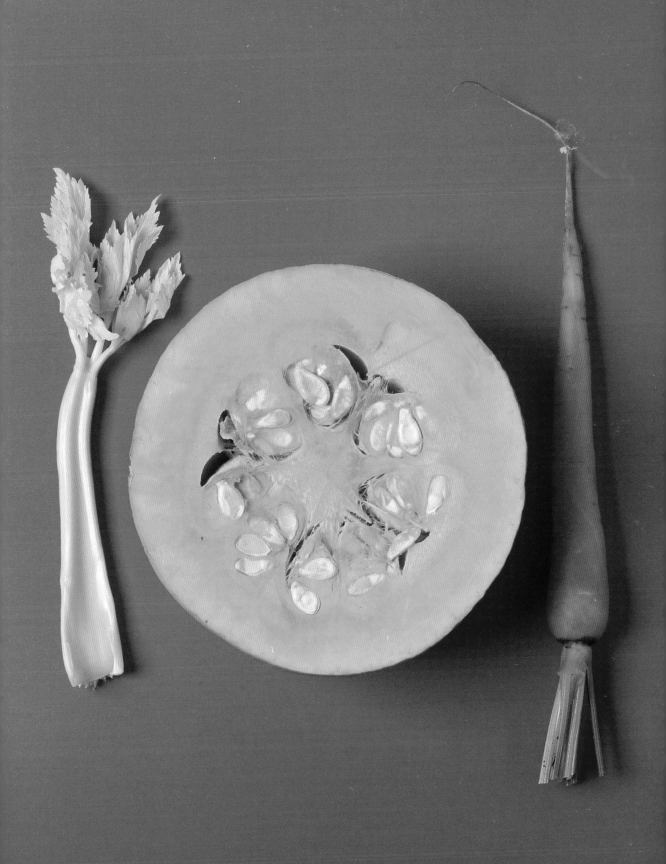

Whatever your starting point, everyone's goal is the same – to eat well. **To eat what your body requires so you can** feel energetic and healthy and go on to enjoy all the good things life has to offer, **leaving behind the fads, hang-ups, guilt, depression, anxiety and debilitating obsession.** Start to eat well, and food begins to have less of a hold over your life, which, after all, is complicated enough. **You eat when you feel hungry, you enjoy what you eat and you feel good afterwards.** You know when to stop, but you don't deny yourself either.

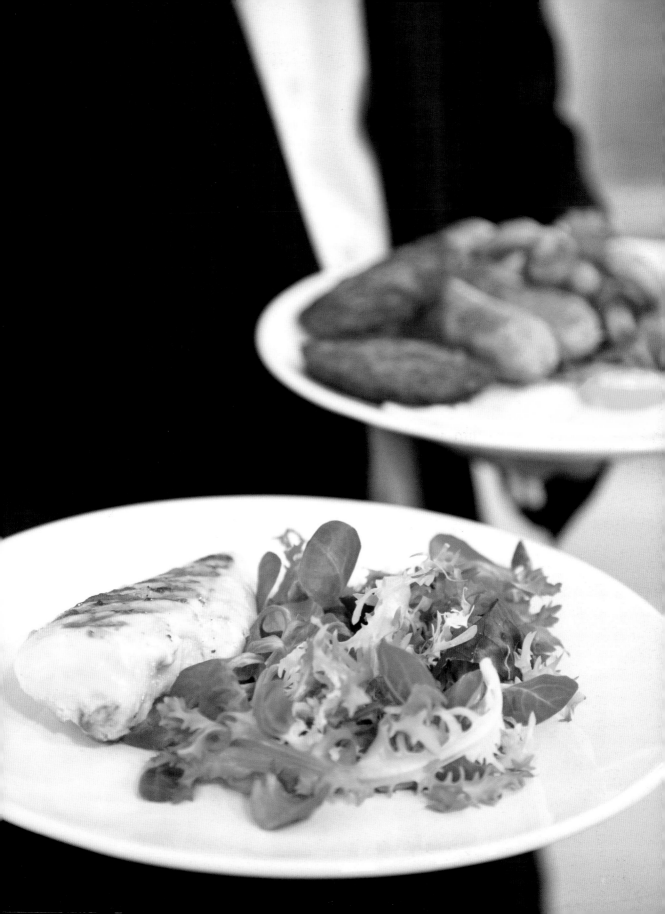

One **for all**

The wonderful thing about our bodies, which makes my life as a doctor somewhat easier, is that we all work in the same way.

We all need the same nutrients to keep functioning. Our age, build, gender and lifestyle determine the amount of energy we need to consume, but that's the only real difference. Tall or heavily built people need more energy – that is, more food – than small, slender ones. As do people constantly on the move, in heavy physical jobs or who have active lifestyles, such as sportspeople or parents of small children. It's rather like comparing a Mini with a Ferrari: they both need petrol for fuel, oil to ensure the engine runs smoothly, water for cooling and brake fluid to stop. But the amounts they use, and the rates at which they use them, will be quite different. It might seem a paradox, but the Supersizes need so much energy just to keep their very large bodies ticking over that their basal metabolic rate (see page 38) can be higher than that of someone who's fit, active and at an ideal weight. So no more blaming a 'slow metabolism'.

There are four main ways to take control of your weight: eat a healthy, balanced diet, have regular mealtimes, eat the right portion sizes for your energy needs and do regular exercise.

Which makes our eating plan easy. Supersize, Superskinny or anywhere in between, you eat roughly the same foods, only the amounts will be different.

We can all enjoy the same healthy and varied foods — no one need deny themselves anything.

But first, before you change anything, I want you to complete a really important exercise (if you haven't already done so) that will help you assess your own eating habits. I want you to take the time to write a food diary of exactly what you currently eat day to day: include everything you eat, how much, and when. Be honest with yourself. Nobody needs to see it. It will help to highlight the areas you need to change. You will be surprised by some of the things your diary reveals.

So, shock horror – the latest diet craze is to eat a normal range of foods supplying you with plenty of carbohydrates, a decent amount of proteins, a small but important amount of fats, and lots of vitamins and minerals. No food group needs to be excluded, and you eat as much as your body needs. No more and no less, according to your body mass and lifestyle.

Reminder. The key to success lies in:
A healthy balance
Regular mealtimes
Portion control
Regular exercise

Eating what comes naturally

1) **First, familiarize yourself with the main food groups:**
★ Carbohydrates
★ Fruit and vegetables
★ Protein (non-dairy protein, meat and vegetarian)
★ Dairy
★ Fats and oils
Aim to eat from these groups every day: where possible, at each meal. The carbohydrate and fruit and vegetable content need to be the largest; fats and oils the smallest – but they need to be there.

2) **If you don't already cook, start to develop your own repertoire of recipes.** (See the next chapter for some fabulous, healthy, easy recipes.) If you do, why not expand your repertoire?

3) **Stop thinking of your favourite foods as 'forbidden'.** That will only make you want more of them. Being in a state of denial is setting yourself up for a binge. But here's an amazing thing. The more you develop your food knowledge and tune in to the needs of your own body, the more you'll find yourself making better food choices. People who improve their diet begin to find, after a while, that they lose their taste for high-fat, high-sugar, high-salt foods and start to drool at the sight of a juicy peach instead. It happens! That greasy meat pie will lose its lustre.

4) **If you are also starting to do some exercise and getting fitter, then your muscles will become much more efficient at burning calories.** As you get fitter, your metabolism will increase. Even at rest, a strong body needs more calories than an unfit one.

Regular mealtimes

Getting into a healthy-eating routine has helped a great many people with eating problems. It puts food in the right place, breaking the obsessive hold it can have. There's a time to eat, and the rest of the time for doing other things. Having a regular eating plan takes your mind off eating and puts your life into perspective. It frees you.

Eating three meals a day is the norm for healthy eating – ideally sitting down at a table and calmly enjoying the occasion, even if it is only for a 10-minute, one-course breakfast. It is also a good time to spend with family, friends and colleagues. Not surprisingly, many business deals are done around a dining table with a good meal. It is well known that in countries where the love of good food is more central to the culture, such as France, Italy and China, there are fewer overweight people. French women famously claim they don't get fat because they eat regularly and well, and don't snack.

Breakfast, lunch and dinner

Have three main meals every day, with four to five hours between each one. Have a light snack or two in between meals if hunger demands it. Plan your eating around your work and include a good break and a meal in the middle of your working day – even if it is no more than a healthy sandwich and a refreshing water-based drink. Your concentration will be recharged and your efficiency improved. A good employer will always insist on proper meal breaks for the workforce to maximize productivity, so regard yourself as the boss of your own one-person workforce and follow suit.

It helps to stick to set times of the day for meals, but a leeway of an hour or so will do no harm, should circumstances arise to delay a meal.

The Five-Point Plan

1. Always eat breakfast, even just a bowl of cereal and a drink

Skipping a meal at this time of day is not a way to lose weight. Quite the opposite. It's a way to make yourself easy prey to a fatty sugary snack-attack mid-morning. If you can't face eating first thing, at least have a cup of tea or glass of hot water, with lemon and a teaspoon of honey, then pack a light sandwich or have a hot milky coffee and a banana when you get to work.

2. Plan your mealtimes and check your food stocks

That means organizing your shopping ahead so you don't run out of essentials such as cereal, milk, juice or bread for toast.

3. Plan a small light snack to have midway between your meals

if you want it. A piece of fruit or home-made muffin (see page 156) is ideal. A high-fat croissant or doughnut in your coffee break will spoil your appetite for lunch and put your routine out of synch, and you'll find yourself grabbing a bag of high-fat crisps or scoffing another cake in the afternoon.

4. Never get in a situation where you feel ravenously hungry —

aim to feel peckish. That way you can look forward to lunch or your evening meal and will enjoy preparing it. It could even improve your culinary skills.

5. And finally, the golden rule, always leave the table feeling you could have eaten just a little bit more

Don't stagger away feeling uncomfortably full, especially at night when you need to wind down for a good sleep. (Bonus: people who have regularized their mealtimes report a great improvement in the quality of their sleep. There is nothing quite so blissful as waking up refreshed after a good night's sleep. And you're more likely to wake up ready for that all-important first thing: breakfast, which ensures a great start to the following day.) Two tips: Eating slowly is one way to help you become aware when you are pleasantly satisfied, not overfull; so don't load up your fork for the next mouthful until you've finished chewing and swallowing the one you've already got. And don't feel you have to eat everything on your plate (or anyone else's) once you've had enough: you are not a human waste-disposal unit!

The truth about **fats**

Fats and oils are the foods highest in calories, weight for weight. But that doesn't mean they aren't good for you. Skin and hair, for example, need fats in order to be healthy, sleek and glossy.

Take butter, which is delicious and natural, free of transfats (see page 140) but high in saturated fat. Use it at room temperature and spread it thinly; allow your toast or crumpet to cool a little before you spread it with butter, so less sinks in; if you like hot buttery vegetables or pasta then add a small knob of butter to the cooking water just before draining to coat lightly – you get the flavour spread over in a thin film. Using preheated heavy-based griddle pans helps meats and fish brown without extra fat or oil. If your intake of fats has been very high and you are working on reducing it, you'll soon be devising your own ways of cutting down without losing flavour.

It is a common misconception that oils are less fattening than butter. In fact, for those number-crunchers among you, butter is less fattening, weight for weight, than oil, because butter contains water. Butter is 82.2 per cent fat (100g = 744 calories); oil is 99.9 per cent fat (100g = 899 calories). However, generally speaking most vegetable oils have lower saturated-fat levels (the fat that leads to higher cholesterol levels) so are deemed to be healthier. Frying a piece of chicken or fish in olive oil will result in more or less the same calories as frying it in butter, but olive oil contains healthier polyunsaturated or monounsaturated fat.

Some reduced-fat products, such as margarine spreads and half-fat crème fraiche, have added water to reduce the calories.

Working out
your **portions**

The number of portions you allocate yourself will depend on how much you have to lose or gain in the first place, and as you near your ideal goal weight or size, these portions should be adjusted accordingly.
Each individual is different, but here is a guide:

★ If you are Supersize and wishing to lose weight you should aim for:
4 portions protein, 10 portions carbohydrates, 4 portions dairy, 10 portions fruit and veg, 3 portions fats, 2 treats a day.

★ If you are Superskinny and wishing to gain weight you should aim for:
3 portions protein, 8 portions carbohydrates, 3 portions dairy, 8 portions fruit and veg, 3 portions fats, 2 treats a day. Alternatively, use these portion guides if you have already reached your ideal weight and simply wish to maintain a healthy and balanced diet.

If you are finding that you are not losing or gaining weight at a rate of 0.5–1 kilo or 1–2 pounds a week, then you may need to increase or decrease these portion amounts. In this way you will find the right amounts that suit your needs. Remember to keep the foods in the same balance as the examples above.
   Any individual who wants an eating plan tailored to them should ask their doctor to refer them to a suitably qualified health professional.

What is a portion?

At the beginning of your new plan, if you have weight-control in mind, get your eye in by weighing a few items such as potatoes or spoonfuls of cereal to get some idea of size. Your portion size doesn't have to be deadly accurate, just near enough. For meat and fish, check pack weights and divide accordingly. This is one of the most common mistakes people make: taking (or being given) portions that are too large. And then eating the lot!

Decide what you like then work out how many portions of each per day you need. For example, if you have a daily allowance of 8 portions of starchy foods you could have 2 slices of bread (for a sandwich or roll), a bowl of cereal for breakfast and pasta or mashed potatoes in the evening. Which all sounds pretty normal and helps with planning your shopping too.

Don't forget to drink. Aim for 6–8 drinks throughout the day, to include tea and coffee. If your aim is to lose weight, use your fruit allowance of 1 juice diluted with sparkling mineral water. A glass of wine or small glass of beer count as 1 portion within your extras. (For more on water and alcohol, see pages 124 and 123.)

Examples of single-portion sizes follow.

1 portion of carbohydrates (starchy foods)

★ 3 heaped tablespoons of wholegrain breakfast cereals or muesli or oats (made into hot porridge) or 1 Weetabix or Shredded Wheat

★ 1 medium slice of wholemeal bread or half a medium pitta, chapati, tortilla wrap, bagel or roll

★ 2 rye crispbreads or 3 rice cakes or 2 oatcakes

★ 1 boiled medium-size potato (about 100g) or 2 smaller new potatoes or half a larger baked potato

★ 2 heaped tablespoons mashed potatoes

★ 2 heaped tablespoons cooked pasta, noodles, rice, couscous, bulghur or pearl barley grains (about 25g uncooked)

★ 1 digestive biscuit, or half a scone or 1 crumpet or Scotch pancake

1 portion of vegetables or fruit

★ 1 cereal bowl of salad

★ 3 heaped tablespoons of cooked, boiled vegetables – fresh, frozen or canned, such as peas, beans, shredded cabbage or corn

★ 1 medium-size salad or plum tomato or 7 cherry tomatoes

★ 1 medium carrot or courgette or leek

★ ¼ small avocado

★ 1 small banana

★ 1 apple or pear or orange or peach

★ 2 small satsumas or 3 plums or 3 apricots

★ 1 kiwi or fistful of strawberries

★ 4 tablespoons of fresh blueberries

★ 1 large slice of melon or pineapple (about 3cm thick)

★ 1 small (150ml) glass fresh unsweetened fruit juice

★ 1 tablespoon of dried fruit, e.g. raisins, cranberries

1 portion of protein

★ 50g (about 1 medium slice) cooked lean beef, pork, lamb, chicken or turkey (without skin) (from a 100g raw portion)

★ 50g (1 small fillet) of oily fish, such as salmon, tuna, mackerel, sardines*

★ 150g white fish fillet, such as cod, haddock, sole, or seafood, such as prawns, mussels, squid*

★ 150g (about 4 tablespoons) Bolognese meat or pasta sauce or chilli con carne

★ 2 free-range eggs (such as an omelette)

★ 150g (4 heaped tablespoons) cooked or canned lentils or pulses or small can baked beans

★ 100g tofu or Quorn

★ 2 tablespoons unsalted nuts or seeds (such as sunflower or pumpkin) or unsalted nut butter

★ 3 tablespoons hummus (70g)

*include fish/seafood twice a week, one of which should be oily fish

1 portion of dairy

★ 1/3 pint or a medium glass (about 200ml) semi-skimmed or soya milk, or 300ml skimmed milk

★ 1 small 125g pot of natural or fruit yogurt or fromage frais or soya dessert

★ 1 small chunk of full-fat cheese, about 25g, the size of a matchbox

★ 2 heaped tablespoons low-fat cheese, e.g. cottage cheese

1 portion of fats and oils

★ 1 teaspoon vegetable oil (inc. olive oil) or fat spread or softened (i.e. room temperature) butter

★ 1 teaspoon mayonnaise or salad cream or ordinary salad dressing

★ 1 teaspoon double cream or crème fraiche or 2 teaspoons reduced-fat crème fraiche or single or soured cream

1 portion of snacks and treats

Some of these may repeat portions above, which is fine, choose either/or.

★ 2 additional pieces of fruit

★ a small pot of low-fat yogurt

★ 1 slice of wholemeal bread with low-fat spread & yeast extract

★ 2 crispbread with 50g/2oz tuna or thinly spread with peanut butter

★ 1 crispbread with 1 level tablespoon hummus

★ 25g/1oz nuts and raisins

★ 1 mini fruit bun, small cereal bar, mini chocolate bar or chocolate biscuit

★ 2 jaffa cakes, or 2 garibaldi biscuits, or 2 fig rolls

★ 1 scoop of plain ice-cream

Alcohol

As ever, moderation in all things. It helps to remember the safe-drinking levels laid down by government advisory bodies, which have categorized alcohol according to units. One unit of alcohol is measured at 10ml and it takes your liver about two hours to cleanse each unit.

Beer (3–4 per cent abv*)	1 unit	½ pint (287ml)	90 cals
Strong beer (6 per cent abv)	2 units	½ pint (287ml)	about 150 cals
Cider dry (5 per cent abv)	1.5 units	½ pint (287ml)	120 cals
Dry white wine (12 per cent abv)	1 unit	small glass (125ml)	90 cals
Red wine (13 per cent abv)	1 unit	125ml	95 cals
Spirits (40 per cent abv)	1 unit	25ml	50 cals

(plus a mixer which could bring it up to 140 calories)

* alcohol by volume

Alcohol spikes your appetite and has you reaching for salty, fatty crisps or salted nuts by the fistful. But our eating plan is not a brutal regime – a little of what you fancy shall be yours, within boundaries. Allow these within your treats/extras allowance:

★ 125ml glass wine – 1 portion (make this last by adding an amount of equal sparkling water)

★ ½ pint lager or bitter or cider – 1 portion

★ 2 measures (2 tbsp) gin, whisky or vodka – 1 portion

Chocolate

Gone are the days when chocolate came in just two colours — dark and milk, consisting mostly of sugar and vegetable fat. Now we are encouraged to seek out high-quality chocolate of 60—75 per cent cocoa solids made from special variety beans from the Americas, Africa and the Indonesian islands. Good chocolate contains antioxidant phenols (also found in red wine and tea) as well as the minerals iron, magnesium, potassium, phosphorous, copper and calcium. It also contains caffeine and has been described as the world's most pleasant antidepressant. Aficionados regard quality chocolate like fine wine, savouring its aroma, bouquet and mouth feel. But there is also sugar and fat in even the best chocolate. So, yes, you can include some chocolate, but stick to the quality brands and have a small square or two, letting it melt slowly on your tongue to savour the full flavour.

Water

Water makes up 60 per cent of our body weight and, although it has no calorific value, it is the most important nutrient we need each day. We can last for much longer without food than we can last without water. In hot weather, we need even more. Sweating helps the body cool down but if we don't drink to replace the lost liquids and mineral salts we might collapse.

In the west, we rarely have water shortages, there is always a good supply of drinking water on tap, and we gulp down billions of litres of bottled mineral water each day. But many of us still don't drink as many liquids as we should, and many more of us don't take enough of our liquids in the form of pure water. Some children never drink water: they have a juicy drink at breakfast, then a fizzy drink at break, another sugary fruit juice for lunch and even more fizzy drinks at home.

Experts suggest we aim to drink 1.5 to 2 litres a day, depending on our size and activity. That's 6–8 medium size (250–300ml) glasses a day. Some of this can be diluted fresh juice. You can also include a mug or two of tea or coffee. Herbal teas can count towards your water quota, as can carbonated mineral water.

Tap or bottle? There's big business in the sale of bottled water and water filters, even though the water that flows from your tap is perfectly safe. The taste will vary – that is personal preference. Tap water will generally be classed as hard or soft depending on mineral deposits. Hard water contains valuable calcium and magnesium, two important minerals. It costs you nothing to keep healthy by drinking tap water in hard-water areas. Check with your water board about your local water hardness. Bottled water in restaurants adds to the price of the meal and is of no benefit.

Diet drinks I've found that some people drink diet drinks as a substitute for a light meal or snack. Some even think the word 'diet' means these drinks help you lose weight. The bottom line is, if you drink a high number of diet drinks each day (more than a can a day) you can be left feeling even more hungry because they have no energy value whatsoever (see page 21). These sorts of drinks may contain caffeine as well, which makes you pee more, and so dehydrates you. If you only ever drink fizzy-type drinks you can end up quite dehydrated, as well as chock full of chemicals.

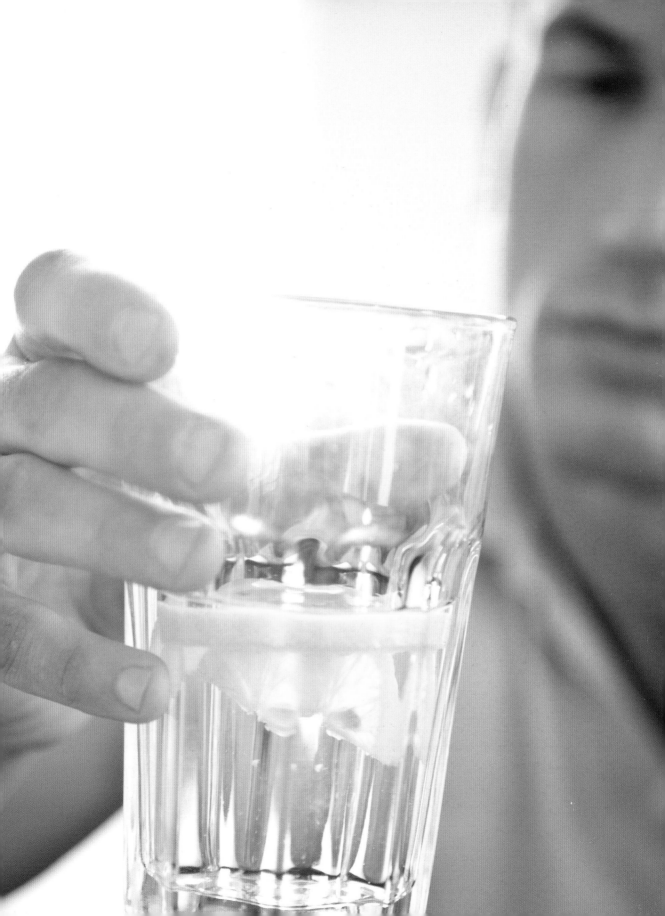

Build your own food plan

The beauty of the eating plan is that by working on portions you can tailor your own plan to your own tastes and needs. If you don't like one food or ingredient, there's no one to make you eat it. Just substitute another from the same food group.

These are the all-important things to remember:

Dairy foods: aim for at least 3 portions a day to ensure you are getting enough calcium. One portion (200ml semi-skimmed milk) can be used in drinks such as teas and coffees.

Breakfast is a must must must: I don't mind saying it again! If you can't eat as soon as you get up, at least start with tea or coffee or even hot water with lemon juice and honey. Then after a shower you should be ready for a bowl of cereal or slice of toast, or a banana or yogurt. If you have to get up a few minutes earlier to factor in breakfast, then do. If you really truly cannot face this vital meal first thing then wait until you almost get to work and stop off to pick up a milky coffee, such as a latte; resist the pastries and have a banana instead.

Do eat your three meals a day, don't skip one and have two bigger meals. Your portions are more beneficial spread out over three meals. Superskinnies who find it hard to eat a normal-size meal at first can eat more frequently. Better to eat six or seven little bites a day than try to eat a full-size 'normal' meal and fail. Choose from the list of snacks on page 128.

Two snacks a day, mid-morning and mid-afternoon, are fine. If you enjoy a hot milky drink at night, try a skinny-milk hot chocolate served in a cup and saucer, which is around half the size of a mug. Supersizers should keep snacks light, such as a piece of fresh fruit or an oatcake or biscuit.

Include starchy foods in each meal. One-third of your foods should come from complex starchy carbohydrates: oats, wholewheat bread, pasta, rice (like brown basmati), quinoa, couscous etc. Snacks, too, can be starchy carbs, but remember not to include sugars in this list. Sugars are simple carbs that do nothing except give you a quick fix of empty energy.

Eat a variety of foods, from all the food groups. One good way to achieve this is to get plenty of colour and texture on your plate. Your total diet plan should take in as many healthy nutrients as possible, and the easiest way to do this is to vary the foods.

Try new tastes. If you have an enquiring palate, the chances are you love good food and the inspiring variety available. Faddy eaters end up with a monotone diet, which is probably why they don't enjoy eating. If this could be you, take time to change the situation, slowly if necessary.

You eat with your eyes

It's a cliché, but it's true. A splodge on a plate is not appealing, especially a greasy splodge. Making your food look good does not require you to do tricks like radish roses or building your food into a tottering stack in the middle of your plate. Simply take a few moments to think about the colours and textures of your meal.

Aim for at least three different colours on your plate. This is also a good way of checking on the variety of foods you eat, a useful indicator of just how balanced your newly formed eating habits are becoming.

Spoon the food on the plate neatly, working from the centre outwards. Finish with a flourish of a small fistful of rocket, watercress or salad, a few halved cherry tomatoes, a trimmed spring onion, a sprinkle of lentil sprouts or some sprigs of parsley or coriander, a spoon of seeds or nuts or even just freshly ground black pepper.

Making your food look great also helps get the gastric juices flowing and aids digestion. Most of all, it will help you appreciate and enjoy what you eat without feeling guilty afterwards.

Snacking

This is the one area that does differ for Supersize and Superskinny. Supersizers need something to keep them going for a couple more hours until the next meal, a stop-gap. Allow two snacks a day, mid-morning and mid-afternoon, in modest portion sizes.

★ 1 large glass of fizzy water or cold iced tea (home-made)
★ 1 small hot-cross bun (without butter)
★ 1 small plain scone
★ 1 crumpet (if you must butter it, let it cool then spread with a teaspoon of butter from your daily portion control)
★ 1 piece of wholemeal or seedy bread toast
★ 2 rice cakes or oatcakes or bread sticks or cream crackers. These could be spread with a little low-fat hummus or thin dabs of Marmite or jam
★ 1 cup of soup
★ 1 small bowl of popcorn, ideally home-made without added fat or sugar
★ About 8 mini pretzels
★ 1 snack pack of raisins and unsalted peanuts
★ 1 carrot or small chunk of cucumber or half a pepper, cut in sticks with half a small pot of raita or reduced-fat hummus
★ 3–4 wine gums or 2 boiled sweets

Superskinnies can have any of the above and also choose from:
★ 1 larger portion of mixed raisins and nuts
★ 1 banana
★ 1 small fistful mixed unsalted nuts, including brazils, hazelnuts, whole almonds and unsalted pistachios
★ A fruity yogurt, not low-fat
★ 1 small milkshake or hot chocolate or café latte
★ 1 small nutty, fruity cereal bar (cut in two if you can't face a whole one)
★ 2 digestive biscuits, even chocolate-coated

Recommended daily portions of food (average)

	Women	Men
	2,000 calories a day	2,500 calories a day
Starchy foods	8	10
Fruit and vegetables	8	10
Dairy	3	4
Meat, fish, proteins	3	4
Fats	3	3
Extras (100 cals each)	2	2

Plate size
Both Supersizers and Superskinnies often find it helpful to use slightly smaller dinner plates. The average plate size is 25—28cm; use a plate of 22—23cm instead so that your portions fill the plate. Supersizers are less inclined to feel cheated and Superskinnies less inclined to feel overwhelmed.

Breakfast ideas

Breakfast is vital. It is probably a good 12 hours since you ate dinner, so you need to 'break your fast', restore energy and get your body back up to operating speed.

Yet it is estimated that around one-third of adults skip this meal each day in the belief it will keep their weight in check. It won't. In fact, it makes you more likely to snack on high-fat sugary foods later on.

Here are some speedy breakfast ideas for when time is limited. For more leisurely, weekend breakfasts, see our recipes on pages 148–159.

★ Choose wholemeal cereals like Bran Flakes, Weetabix, Shredded Wheat etc. Many people are rediscovering the joy of old-fashioned porridge, updated with fast cooking in the microwave in under 5 minutes. Oats are high in soluble fibre, the type that helps remove 'bad' cholesterol from your blood. If you like porridge sweet, instead of a heavy sprinkling of sugar, drizzle with a little honey or maple syrup or add a spoonful of raisins. Watch out for sugary granolas or cereals described as 'clusters of grains' because they are likely to be high in sugar: read the labels.

★ For an Australian breakfast, slice a fresh peach, small mango or an apple (or all three) on top of your cereal and mix with natural yogurt instead of milk. Try muesli softened with some apple juice. Or make smoothies (see page 159) of two or three of your favourite fruits blended with milk.

Out to **lunch**

★ Pack your own sandwiches, varying the breads and fillings (see recipes on pages 166 and 168), but steer clear of ready-made sandwich fillings and coleslaw, which are high in fats (such as in mayo) and salt.

★ Buy lean meat or opt for tuna, sardines and hummus (reduced fat if you are losing weight).

★ For a treat, have smoked salmon and rocket sandwiches, or a brown bagel spread with low-fat soft cheese and salmon.

★ If you want to cut down on bread, or get bored of it, choose other starchy food instead. Take in a box of grain salad using couscous or bulghur wheat as a base mixed with lentils or chickpeas, chopped tomatoes, peppers, cucumber and grated courgette.

★ Pasta, rice, lentils, beans, peas and other pulses and grains, mixed together in various combinations with a light dressing of olive oil and vinegar or lemon juice, are perfectly balanced nutritionally. Or take a pot of 2–3 tablespoons of hummus to work with you, and some fingers of carrot, pepper and cucumber, plus sliced pitta bread.

★ Hot soup in a flask is perfect for winter, and chilled home-made gazpacho or creamy cucumber and yogurt make delicious lunches in summer.

Food retail
therapy

Coming home hungry to an empty fridge after a long day at work is asking for trouble. It's too easy to reach for the phone and call up the pizza man. Instead, spend a few minutes working out menus for at least three or four evening meals ahead, especially for the days when you know you could be late home. (And while you're at it, bin those junk-mail takeaway menus too.) Planning doesn't have to be down to the last potato or carrot. Just the main part of each meal – whether you will have chops one day, salmon fillet the next, chicken breasts and so on.

Avoid buying ready meals regularly, as they are often very high in calories and fats. (And expensive too.) Instead keep them for an occasional treat, and then choose from a healthy range ready meal. If you live on your own, check the pack for a single portion size. Too often they serve two.

Ignore the BOGOF (Buy One Get One Free) deals. Unless it is for two packs of chicken or salmon or fresh vegetables. Meat and fish you can freeze for later.

Practise or brush up on your basic cooking skills. Use chapter 8 of this book. When you've tried all the recipes you want, there are a host of quick and easy cookbooks out there. And the major supermarkets all offer free recipe cards, a good proportion of which are healthy, lean dishes with helpful 'What to buy' lists included. They couldn't make it easier for you.

Buy a fridge magnet and stick your rough menu on the fridge door. It will allow you to anticipate what's for supper each evening and look forward to it. Vary the main protein element, making sure you eat lean chicken and beef, pork or lamb plus fish twice a week. And try a veggie main meal once in a while, using pulses, Quorn or tofu; it could be quite a pleasant experience. An aubergine and potato moussaka makes a delicious, lighter change from a meat-based one, for example.

Discover farmers' market shopping. More and more town centres are hosting local farmers' markets where small food-producers, many of whom follow organic or ethical farming methods, display their freshly harvested produce. Fresh vegetables, fruits, farmhouse cheeses, breads, pickles, fish and meats all make food shopping a pleasure. Talk to the stallholders and share their enthusiasm for good food honestly produced. Learn to cook and eat with the seasons and soon you'll find the pleasure of eating well-balanced meals, just like our forebears did.

Try a new food occasionally, even if you find you don't like it. At least you've tried to increase your food horizons. If you feel your palate has been somewhat limited, then work your way through the alphabet of foods. Start with aubergines, asparagus and artichokes and work your way through to fennel, squashes, sweet potato, scallops or venison. Try eating familiar foods in new exciting ways. Griddle vegetables instead of boiling them, or steam them Chinese-style with ginger, garlic and soy sauce. Roast sweet potatoes are a great healthy alternative to roast potatoes (see page 213).

Make sure your storecupboard and fridge are well stocked so you can always rustle up a quick meal (see pages 134–137).

Food markets are great places to learn about new foods and even how to prepare them.

Storecupboard
basics

★ Cans of pulses, choose from mixed beans, chickpeas, lentils or flageolet or kidney beans

★ Capers in brine

★ Stoned black olives

★ Reduced-fat tomato pasta sauce

★ Cartons of sieved tomatoes or cans of chopped tomatoes

★ Tuna in water or olive oil

★ Sardines in tomato sauce

★ Sweetcorn in water

★ Seed and nut mixes

★ Jars of char-grilled artichokes, sun-dried tomatoes, chillies and peppers, but if packed in oil, pat dry before use

★ Jars of pickled beetroots, chutney and relishes

★ Stock cubes or bouillon stock powder

★ Packets of rice (especially brown basmati, and Arborio for risottos), pasta, couscous, bulgur wheat

★ Low-salt Kikkoman soy sauce (the best naturally brewed sauce)

★ Canned fruit in fruit juice

★ Wholegrain breakfast cereals and oats

★ Sea salt, black peppercorns, dried oregano (other leafy herbs, such as parsley, coriander, thyme, tarragon and chives are best bought fresh), curry powder (Indian and Thai), ground cinnamon, cumin and coriander

Keep in the **fridge** or **freezer**

★ Freshly grated parmesan cheese (it stays crumbly when frozen)
★ Fresh vegetables in packs and fresh pasta often have long Use By dates so they will keep for up to a week in the fridge
★ Baby new potatoes, sweet potatoes, turnips and parsnips will all store in the lower fridge vegetable drawer, as will peppers, onions, fennel bulbs and cabbage
★ Spring onions are great: they can be quickly chopped and don't make you cry
★ Tubes of garlic, ginger puree, tomato puree
★ Tubs of reduced-fat crème fraiche (these last a week when opened)
★ Pesto (use a tablespoon per meal for two)
★ Packs of fresh herbs – such as parsley, coriander, thyme, tarragon, chive – any of which can be scissor-snipped straight into sauces, pan-fries, salads in bountiful amounts; they are full of vitamins and minerals as well as being delicious
★ In the freezer: frozen vegetables, especially peas

Superfast
storecupboard meals

These meal ideas use food from the storecupboard or freezer and/or leftovers from the fridge. They all take 10 minutes or less.

Pasta for one

Boil your favourite pasta. Drain and toss back into the pan. Stir in 1 small can tuna (drained and flaked) + 1 small can chopped tomatoes + pinch dried herbs + 3 tbsp frozen peas + 1 tsp garlic puree + 1 tsp capers and/or black olives. Season and reheat until it bubbles then serve with a light sprinkling of freshly grated parmesan.

Lentil and egg kedgeree for one

Using cold leftover rice, about 1 small mugful (or try a pack of plain pre-cooked basmati), reheat in a non-stick saucepan until hot with ½ can lentils + 2 spring onions, chopped + 1 tsp curry paste + 1 (of 2) chopped hard-boiled egg + 2–3 tbsp frozen green beans + small knob of butter or tsp olive oil. Peel and quarter the remaining egg and serve on top.

Bacon chilli for one

Snip and dry-fry 2 rashers bacon in a non-stick pan then mix in 1 small mugful cold leftover rice (or 1 pack pre-cooked rice) + 1 small can red kidney beans + 1 small can chopped tomatoes + chilli sauce to taste topped with 1 tsp reduced-fat crème fraiche and snipped fresh coriander.

Anchovy and broccoli spaghetti for one

Boil spaghetti and for the last 2 minutes drop in 3–4 small frozen broccoli florets then drain. Take ½ can of anchovies and snip in along with 1 tsp garlic puree. Mix and top with 1 tbsp freshly grated parmesan.

Chowder for two

Heat together 1 can lobster bisque or soupe de poisson + 3 tbsp canned sweetcorn + 1 cooked medium potato, finely chopped + 1 tomato, chopped + 2 spring onions, chopped + 1 mug stock and skimmed milk + 1 small can clams, drained. Simmer for 2 minutes then serve.

Warm tuna and beetroot salad for two

Boil 4 baby new potatoes then slice. Mix 1 medium can tuna + 2 pickled beetroots, chopped + ½ can white beans, drained + 2 eggs, hard-boiled and quartered. Toss with warm new potatoes and 1–2 tbsp vinaigrette dressing (see page 166).

Reading labels

The more food we prepare ourselves from fresh raw ingredients, the better. However, we need to know our way around supermarket foods too. To understand what we are consuming, we need to be adept at reading labels.

Nutritionists have established what are known as RDAs (Recommended Daily Amounts) of important vitamins and minerals, which we need to make sure we eat enough of. They have also established GDA (Guideline Daily Allowances), especially geared towards nutrients we tend to eat too much of. All food manufacturers must by law now print a minimum of the basic nutritional figures relevant to the product on their packs. Figures for the relevant nutrients for each product are listed per 100g (so you can compare like with like) and sometimes per suggested portion. In addition, some manufacturers give an outline of the daily requirements for 'average' men and women in terms of energy, fats and carbohydrates. You don't have to memorize all the facts and figures, just be aware of the outlines.

We all need energy to keep going. This will be listed as kcals (or kilocalories, but what in day-to-day speech are just called 'calories') or even kJ (kilo Joules, after the British scientist who devised the more accurate energy measure).

★ Carbohydrate figures will be divided into complex starchy carbs and simple sugars.
★ Proteins – from meat, fish, dairy or vegetables.
★ Fats are divided into two categories: saturated fats (the animal-based hard fats) and unsaturated fats – polyunsaturated or monounsaturated (the healthier vegetable-based ones).
★ You might also get figures for EFAs – that is, Essential Fatty Acids, such as omega 3 and 6.
★ There will also be figures for fibre and salt, including pure sodium.

If a manufacturer is proud of his nutrients he is going to make sure you know about it. And conversely if he prefers not to draw your attention to the lack of a nutrient, its absence will speak volumes.

So a nutritional label gives you a quick outline of how healthy or not the food is. In addition you should get a box giving you the daily inclusive nutrients for men and women, and, if there is space on the pack, a good manufacturer will list the percentage that particular portion of food will be of the Guideline Daily Allowance (GDA).

But remember the figures are for average adults.

GDAs per day	Women	Men
Calories	2,000	2,500
Fat	70g	95g
of which saturates	20g	30g
Salt	6g	6g
Total sugars	90g	120g

Flavour enhancers

Processed food is actually very bland to start with because it is not cooked in the same way we cook at home. The act of cooking involves browning and simmering and grilling or frying, all of which brings out the best of natural flavour. Browning meat or onions in a hot pan, for example, caramelizes the natural juices. But processed food is often just a mixture of prepared foods all bundled into a giant cooking pot, sealed and brought up to a high temperature. Left like that it would be dull and no one would enjoy it or buy it again.

So manufacturers look for ways of adding flavour. Salt improves flavour, but add too much and the food becomes inedible (not to mention unhealthy). There are a number of flavour enhancers that don't have a flavour in themselves but when combined with other foods make the foods taste better. The best known, monosodium glutamate (MSG), was discovered in Japan over a hundred years ago when a scientist extracted a chemical from seaweed called glutamate and found that while it was tasteless, it enhanced other flavours. It has found its way into many foods, from those you might expect, such as soy sauce, to others less obvious. Some people feel they have a reaction (such as a headache, or a feeling of being unwell) to it in high quantities.

There are many other permitted flavour enhancers, produced from a variety of natural ingredients such as bark, vegetable proteins, gluten, even sardines. They have long chemical names often ending with the letters –ate which should give you a clue if you are examining the tiny label print. Asthmatics and those sensitive to aspirin may be advised to avoid flavour enhancers. Hydrolyzed vegetable proteins broken down into amino acids are also used as flavour enhancers.

Transfats

'Transfats' has become another 'beware' buzz word placed firmly on the side of 'baddie' fats (the ones that not only increase levels of bad LDL blood cholesterol but also, it seems, reduce the levels of the good HDL cholesterol).

Vegetable oils are low in saturated fats and higher in healthy monounsaturates and polyunsaturates. Vegetable oils are naturally liquid at room temperature, which makes them tricky to use in cooking and baking. To make vegetable oils solid they undergo a process known as hydrogenation. This is how we get tubs of soft margarines and olive oil spreads. Research then found that the very process of hydrogenation – of solidifying these healthy vegetable fats – altered them to raise the levels of bad LDLs and lessen the good HDLs. Some researchers even said transfats were worse for our health than saturated fats.

It is quite a bewildering disappointment. What we once thought of as a way of enjoying spreadable, creamy fats can now cause us the same problems as if we were eating animal fats such as butter, lard and suet. We are in effect almost back to square one. Some food experts now say let's eat butter anyway, but in small healthy amounts, along with liquid healthy oils. And food manufacturers who used to use transfats are now looking to substitute them with other cleverly composed healthy vegetable fats and declare their products 'transfats free'. As always, check the label.

Salt

The oldest food preservative in the world, and a precious item from prehistory to today. We must have some salt in our diet for various vital bodily functions; we will die without it.

But we can also have too much of it. Our bodies need only around 6g a day: a teaspoonful. (For children it is just 2–3g a day, depending on age.) Which sounds a lot if you think of it solely as what you sprinkle over food, but in fact you are likely to be taking in unknown amounts of 'hidden salt' in processed foods, and then there's the salt you add in cooking too.

People who eat very little processed food can keep tabs on their salt intake. But most of us eat some processed food each day. Bread has it, as do breakfast cereals, most butter, cheese, biscuits (sweet and savoury), then the more obvious foods such as crisps, canned soups and sauces, fish fingers, ketchup, mayonnaise, smoked fish and ham, not to mention bacon, prawns and soy sauce (lots there), and that's before we come on to the heavily processed foods like takeaway burgers, pizzas and fried chicken.

Experts believe three-quarters of our salt intake comes in processed food, which means most of us will have already exceeded our RDA before we even add any salt at home. A number of manufacturers have reduced some of their salt levels but reducing from a lot still leaves quite a bit.

On a food label, salt may be listed as sodium. This is because the real name for salt is sodium chloride. But it's the sodium part that causes the problem. So if a food label lists only sodium, don't be fooled into thinking it means salt. Multiply the sodium figure by 2.5 to give you the full amount.

Another way of checking salt levels is to look at the Traffic Light labels on the front of packs: red = high in salt, amber = all right in moderation, green = low in salt.

So aim to choose foods that are mostly amber or green, opting for mostly green if you know you have to cut back. There are some who think sea salt is healthier – take that with a pinch of salt. It isn't healthier – but it just tastes better, so you probably use a little less.

Reducing salt levels to around 6g a day will certainly help to cut deaths caused by strokes, heart attacks, high blood pressure and kidney disease. That's a saving of around 35,000 premature deaths a year in the UK.

Sugars

Every teaspoon of highly refined sugar supplies around 20 calories, and nothing else. So if you have two spoons of sugar in four or five cups of tea or coffee a day, that's 100 calories straight off. Add to that any biscuits, muffins, cakes, puddings, ice-creams or sweets you might eat, and it can make for an unhealthy amount of sugar. Then add on the sugar in products you weren't expecting to contain sugar: most cereals (even the so-called healthy mueslis), baked beans, tomato pasta sauces, ketchup, canned cooking sauces, drinks and squashes – the list goes on.

The most popular and easily available form of sugar is sucrose, which we call 'sugar' (the granulated, caster and icing sugars), made from sugar beet and sugar cane. Nutritionally there is no difference between the two. Then there are fruit-derived sugars called fructose (honey is the most widely available). The other sugars you may find listed on packaging are lactose (from milk), maltose (from malt) and glucose (the simplest form of sugar; it's also the sugar our food is broken down into during digestion).

This is useful to know when you come to read labels on products; they will all be listed as 'sugars' under the carbohydrate figures. They all have roughly the same energy value (calories) but because fructose is sweeter you can use less. Fructose also has a lower GI value (see page 106) and takes longer to digest and be absorbed into our bloodstream. It can therefore help diabetics control their sugar intake more effectively than high-GI sucrose. The other sugars may have minute amounts of trace elements of minerals (contributing to flavour and colour), but in essence they are still high in energy and not much else.

Apart from the danger to our body shape of too much sugar, there is the danger it poses to our dental health. Sugar remains in our mouths after we have swallowed sweet foods, hanging around the tooth enamel, turning into plaque (the furry film you feel at the end of the day) and being fed on by bacteria, leading to tooth decay. When you eat sugary foods of any kind, find an opportunity to swill out your mouth with fresh water afterwards.

Cleaning teeth twice a day helps to remove plaque but in between meals dentists often encourage us to chew sugar-free gum, because the action of chewing releases saliva in the mouth, helping keep tooth-decaying bacteria in check. Most sugar-free chewing gums contain either sorbitol, a natural extract from stone fruits and berries, or xylitol, originally derived from birch trees in Finland. So that should solve the mystery about why dentists tell us to cut down on sugars for our dental health but chewing gum still tastes sweet.

Artificial sweeteners

From the late 19th century onwards, scientists discovered other substances that tasted sweet but contained very few calories. These were labelled as artificial sweeteners and their level of sweetness was measured against commonly available sugar (sucrose). Saccharin was the first of these, developed in 1878. It was three hundred times the sweetness of sugar, but had a number of downsides, not least a bitter aftertaste and concerns about being involved in causing cancers.

Common sugar (sucrose) is high in calories and gives us nothing except quick spurts of energy and, if we are not careful with our dental hygiene, bad teeth. So food manufacturers continue to spend billions in research projects to give us safe low-to-zero calorie alternatives that won't cause dental problems or contribute to weight gain. Artificial sweeteners do have a calorie value but, because they are hundreds of times sweeter than sugar, weight for weight, we only need, and should only use, a tiny amount, making them almost calorie-free. Consequently, artificial sweeteners will not raise the carbohydrate 'of which sugars' figures in a nutritional information box by any more than a tiny amount. However, this is not a perfect solution, because these new sweeteners have other side effects. They are excreted rather than digested and, in some cases, an excess of these substances can lead to diarrhoea or constipation. Much of the ongoing research into sugar and sweeteners is associated with research into diabetes.

There are three main sweeteners used in the food-processing business and they have their supporters and critics. All have been given an 'E' number, which you should find on the back of packs.

Aspartame (E951) is 180 times sweeter than sugar with just 4 calories per gram. It is commonly used in thousands of foods and soft drinks around the world. Common trademark names are Canderel and NutraSweet, and you may also find it used in sugar-free chewing gum. You can use it sprinkled lightly over fruit or cereals or in hot tea and coffee but it is not suitable for cooking as it becomes bitter upon heating. There has been a growing chorus of voices raised against aspartame, based on claims that it is addictive and, in certain cases, can cause health problems. Those who eat or drink large quantities of food containing it claim they suffer withdrawal symptoms such as headaches and aching limbs when they try to cut down.

Acesulfame K (the K stands for potassium, E950) is 200 times sweeter than sugar and widely used in processed foods and drinks. It is frequently used in combination with other sweeteners, often aspartame, but unlike aspartame it can be used in cooking without becoming bitter-tasting, and is often combined with other sweeteners because of its 'sugar-like' flavour.

Sucralose (E955) is the sweetest sweetener at more than 600 times that of sugar, and was developed in conjunction with the sugar giants Tate and Lyle. It is sold under the Splenda brand name and can be used in cooking and baking. As it is so sweet only a tiny, tiny amount is needed to take the place of sugar, so it can be marketed as a 'no-calorie' sweetener. It is sold in light fluffed-out packs containing fillers to give it volume.

At this point it is useful to remember this rule of thumb:
★ the fewer processed foods and artificial ingredients you eat, and the more fresh meals prepared from natural ingredients you consume instead, the better for your general health.

chapter eight

recipes for life

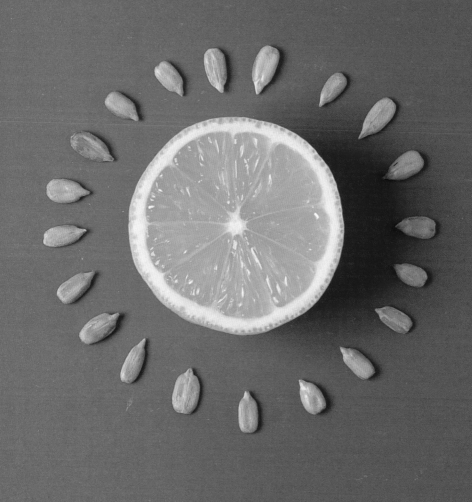

It's funny how we all worry about what we eat between Christmas and New Year. We'd be better off thinking instead about what we eat between New Year's Day and Christmas.

Good simple food you make yourself from healthy ingredients you have chosen is better than anything you'll find ready-made in a packet in a supermarket or on the back of a fast-food delivery scooter. Not only does it taste better – try it and see – but it's also healthier and often cheaper too. Developing a repertoire of quick, easy and great-tasting recipes is one of the keys to eating well, and feeling great, for life.

If you are maintaining a steady weight – neither losing weight, nor gradually allowing yourself to gain weight – you can enjoy these recipes exactly as they are, with or without add-on extras, whatever you fancy. If you are trying to lose weight, however, follow the Lean Tips, measure portions accurately, use semi-skimmed milk, use a spritzer to oil pans, don't automatically spread butter on bread, and so on.

Most of all, enjoy food: you are meant to. Rather than waking up thinking: I mustn't eat this or that today, focus your mental energy on a positive – remember that, every single day, you get to choose from an array of wonderful foods, with which you can create meals you will love. And your body will love you for it.

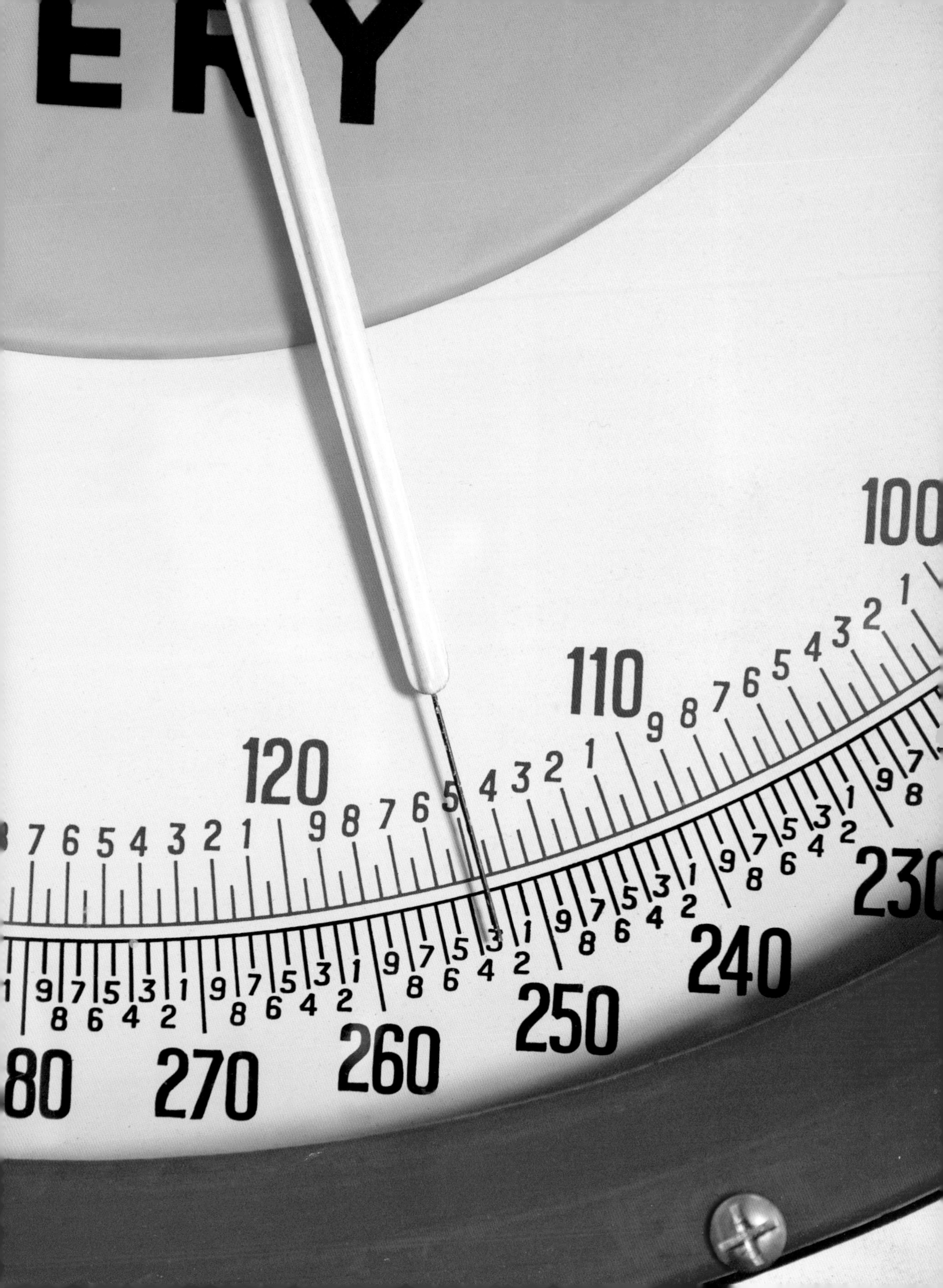
ERY
100
110
120
230
240
250
260
270

muesli

Make a batch of your own sugar-free muesli each week and store it in a large glass jar. Vary the nuts, seeds and fruits to taste. Toasting the base adds extra flavour and crunch. Serve with milk or soak briefly in a little cold water and top with natural yogurt and sliced fresh fruit. Perfect for Superskinnies.

Makes 7 portions, enough for a week

3 tbsp almond flakes or hazelnuts or pecans, roughly chopped

3 tbsp desiccated coconut

3 tbsp sunflower seeds

3 tbsp pumpkin seeds

2 tbsp linseeds

200g jumbo porridge oats

1 tsp ground cinnamon or nutmeg

2 Weetabix, crumbled

50g of two of the following: raisins, dried cranberries or blueberries, snipped dried apricots, dates or apple rings

1 Heat the oven to 180°C/Gas 4. Toss the nuts, coconut and seeds together in a bowl to mix then spread out on a baking tray. Toast for 10 minutes, stirring once or twice.

2 Remove and cool. Mix into the oats, sprinkle with the spice then crumble over the Weetabix and tip into a storage jar. Add the fruits of choice, screw on the lid and shake well. Use within a week.

french toast

Perfect for breakfast or brunch, and a good way of stretching one egg to feed two. Use white or light brown bread or try a sunflower-seed loaf, but not a heavy wholemeal. Serve dusted with icing sugar (for Supersizers) or drizzle lightly with maple syrup (for Superskinnies). Lovely with strawberries or sliced peach, or both.

Serves 2

1 free-range medium egg
2 tbsp milk
2 thick slices bread
1 tbsp or 2 spritzes olive oil
1–2 tsp icing sugar (for Supersizers) or 2 tbsp maple syrup
  (for Superskinnies)
pinches of ground cinnamon
sliced strawberries or peaches, to serve

1 Beat the egg well in a shallow bowl then add the milk. If the bread has thick crusts trim them off, then cut each slice diagonally.
2 Heat a medium-sized non-stick frying pan until you feel a good heat rising and add a scant tablespoon of oil, swirling it around the pan, or give the hot pan 2 spritzes with your spray bottle.
3 Dunk the bread slices quickly in the egg on both sides and place in the pan. Cook 2–3 minutes each side on a medium heat until golden brown and crisp. Remove to two plates.
4 Tap the icing sugar through a fine sieve over the toasts or drizzle with the syrup, then sprinkle with the cinnamon. Serve with sliced fruit.

Lean Tips
Fill a pump–action spritzer bottle with olive or vegetable oil. Use it to get the best coverage of the pan with the least amount of oil when frying.

Lighten your sugar intake with icing sugar. It tastes sweeter because it dissolves more quickly on your tongue and you use less as a consequence.

supersizesuperskinny

149

fruit–tea fruit salad

Wake your taste buds up in the morning with these fresh, tangy flavours. Choose a mixture of fresh and dried fruits and soak in your favourite fruit tea. Perk it up with cranberries and aromatic whole spices in winter or fresh berries in summer. Keeps for several days in the fridge. Great for Supersizers. Superskinnies can add sliced fresh dates, bananas and chopped nuts, and top with a dollop of Greek yogurt mixed with a teaspoon of honey.

Serves 4

6 dried apricots
4 stoned prunes or dried figs
2–4 slices dried peach
1 fruit or Earl Grey tea bag
1 pink grapefruit or a large orange

In winter
1 cinnamon stick and 4 cloves, optional
1 tbsp dried cranberries, optional

In summer
small handful fresh raspberries or blueberries, optional

1 Snip the apricots, prunes or figs and peach slices in half. Cover with about 300ml boiling water and add the tea bag. Bring to the boil and simmer for 5 minutes, then take off the heat, add the whole spices, if using, and set aside to cool.
2 Meanwhile, cut the peel and pith from the grapefruit or orange by removing the ends first, then standing the fruit upright on a board and cutting off the peel in strips. Halve the fruit, then slice into half-moons.
3 Remove the tea bag and spices from the dried fruits. Add the dried cranberries, if using, and the grapefruit or orange slices, along with any juices from the chopping board. Chill for a good 2 hours or overnight.
4 Serve chilled, scattered with the fresh berries, if using.

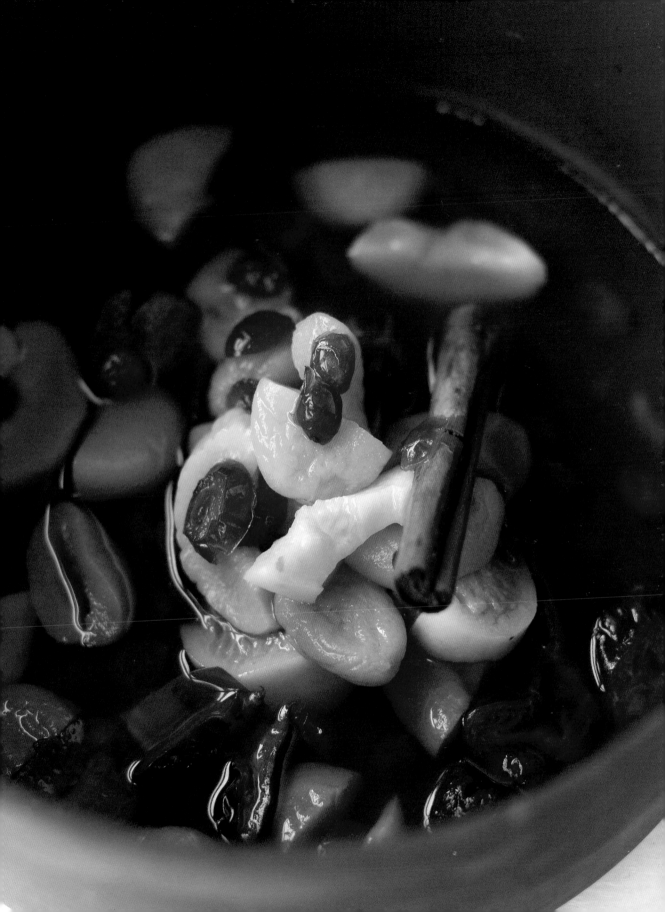

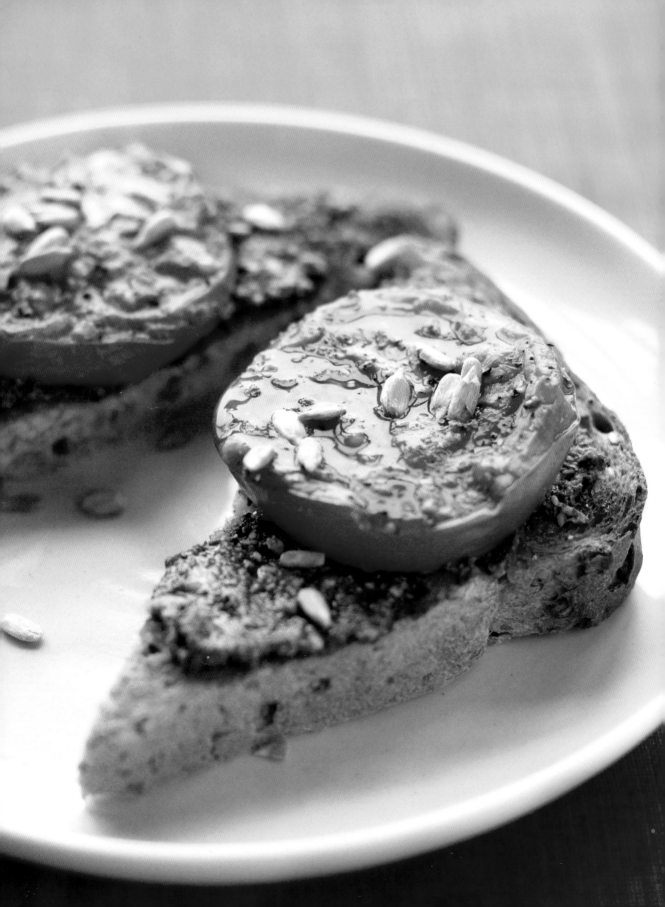

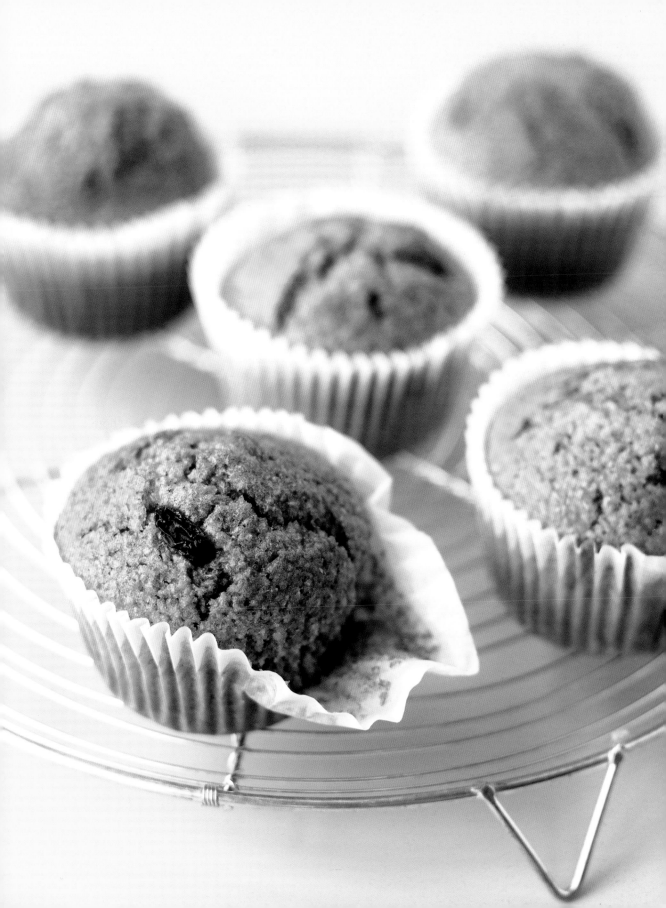

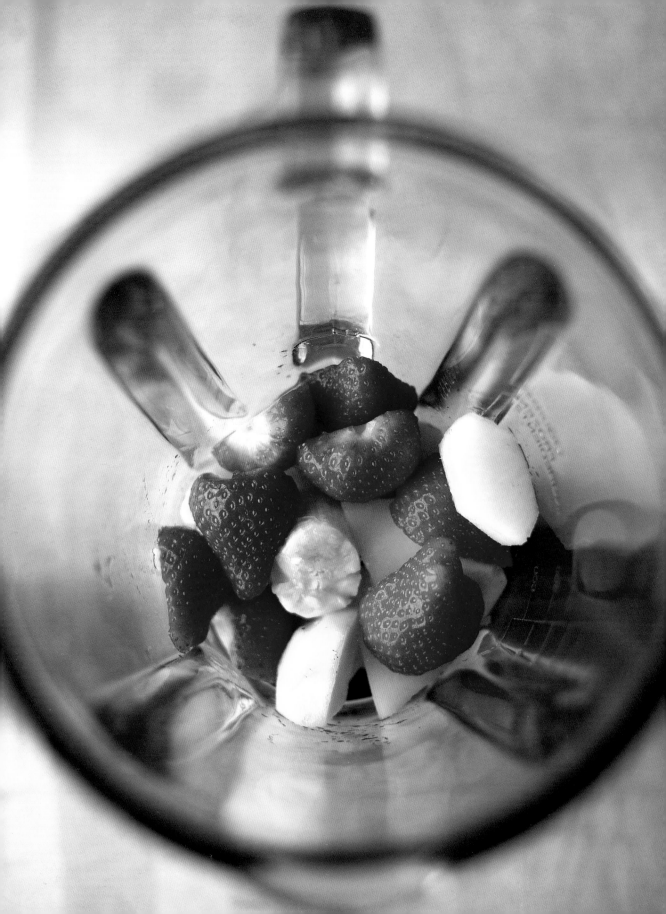

fruity smoothies

Anyone who finds it hard to eat breakfast should try a smoothie. Choose 2 or 3 fruits and whiz them together, with tangy buttermilk or skimmed milk added for extra protein. Satisfying and effortless breakfast-in-a-glass.
Serves 1

Choose 2 or 3 fruits from this list
1 small banana, just ripe
1 small pear
$\frac{1}{2}$ dessert apple, core removed
1 large plum, stoned
small handful seedless grapes
small cup chopped mango or fresh pineapple
small cup raspberries or blueberries
3 or 4 strawberries
$\frac{1}{2}$ papaya (seeded and peeled)

about 100ml skimmed milk or buttermilk, chilled
dustings of freshly ground nutmeg or cinnamon

1 Prepare the fruits of your choice and whiz to a thick blend in a liquidizer or processor. If you are using skimmed milk or buttermilk, whiz it in for a few seconds for a lighter and more creamy result.
2 Pour into a tall glass, over ice cubes if you like, and grate over some nutmeg or dust with cinnamon.

panzanella: tuscan tomato, olive and bread salad

A traditional Italian country salad that is the definition of effortless healthy eating. Ideal for lunch boxes too.

Serves 1

1 thick slice rustic bread
1 large beef tomato or 2 smaller plum tomatoes, halved or thinly sliced
about 4 large fresh basil leaves, torn
a few thin slices of red onion
1 tbsp extra virgin olive oil (or spritz to reduce the amount)
1 tbsp balsamic vinegar
about 4 pitted black olives, sliced

Lean Tip
Take 2 pump-action spritzer bottles, one filled with olive oil and one with balsamic vinegar, and use them to spray salad leaves. You use less dressing and the leaves are coated more evenly.

1 Break up the bread into bite-size pieces then dunk quickly into a bowl of cold water and squeeze gently. Place in a shallow bowl or food container.
2 Place the tomatoes, basil and onion on top and sprinkle or spritz with the oil and vinegar. Season, cover and leave for about an hour for the juices to sink into the bread, then stir roughly together. Scatter with the olives and serve.

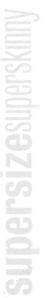

supersizesuperskinny

toast and toasties

A slice or two of hot toast is a good healthy snack base as long as you keep the fat content light and the toppings lean and healthy. Vary the bread base with wholemeal, sourdough, granary and seeded breads, and baguettes, bagels and rolls. Spread lightly with butter if you want to, but why not learn to love fresh toast without fat, especially if you use soft toppings like a poached egg, squashy tomatoes or even baked beans.

Toppings/toasties serve 1

Creamy mushroom and parma ham
Slice a large portobello mushroom. Heat a non-stick frying pan until hot and spritz once or trickle in 1 tsp oil. Add the mushroom slices, cooking until they brown, then flip over, season, add 1–2 tbsp water, cover and lower the heat slightly and cook for 1–2 more minutes. Stir in 2 tsp reduced-fat crème fraiche and pile on to the toast. Top with a slice of parma or serrano ham.

Scrambled egg and salmon
Beat a free-range egg in a cup with 1–2 tbsp milk and seasoning. Heat a small non-stick saucepan until hot and spritz once or drizzle in 1 tsp oil. Tip in the egg and stir briskly to scramble then scoop immediately back into the cup so it does not overcook. Toast a muffin or bagel, pile on the egg and arrange a slice or two of smoked salmon and a small handful of rocket on top. Grind with extra pepper and serve.

Red bean and garlic cheese
Mash 2–3 tbsp canned red kidney beans with 1 tbsp reduced-fat soft garlic cheese using a fork. Add a good pinch of paprika and ground cumin and pile on hot toast.

Brie and mushroom toasties
Place lightly greased bread in the base of a sandwich maker, a slice of brie (about 20g) on top, and pile on 2–3 sliced mushrooms. Season, top with another bread slice, press together and cook.

fillings for pittas

Cut pittas in half, then open up carefully using your fingers to create little pockets. Fill with crisp lettuce and vegetables in bite-size pieces. These make ideal packed lunches: take the filling in a box and keep the bread separate, then make up on the spot for an instant lunch.

Fillings serve 1 (1 pitta)

Chickpea and feta salad

In a bowl, mix 1 sliced or chopped medium-sized tomato, a short length of cucumber cut into slices or chopped, 1 chopped spring onion, 2 tbsp crumbled feta cheese, a large pinch of mint or dill and 2 tbsp canned chickpeas. Spoon into both pitta halves.

Egg and rocket salad

Make scrambled egg with 1 egg and a little milk, cooked in 1 tsp olive oil (see page 165). Season, then mix in a pinch of cumin or mild curry powder and a chopped spring onion. Stuff some rocket, watercress or baby salad leaves into both pitta halves and spoon in the egg.

Chinese chicken

Use ready-cooked Chinese-flavoured chicken breast, 50g per serving. Pull into shreds, moisten with 2 tsp home-made low-fat vinaigrette and mix with sliced red pepper, shredded cos or little gem lettuce (or Chinese leaves) and a good handful of bean sprouts. Stuff into the pitta halves.

Low-fat vinaigrette
Put 4 tbsp olive oil in a screw-top jar and add 2 tbsp wine vinegar, 100ml water, 2 tsp French mustard, 2 tsp clear honey, a good pinch of salt, black pepper and dried mixed herbs. Screw the lid on tightly and shake well. Makes about 200ml, enough for 8 salads. Transfer to a pump-action spritzer bottle to get really good salad coverage.

supersizesuperskinny

baked potato fillings

Allow a medium-sized potato per portion (about 150–200g). Score the top in a cross then bake in the oven for 40 minutes at 180°C/Gas 4, or microwave for 5–7 minutes on full then let stand for 3 minutes. Push up from the base to open up. Choose one filling per potato.

Fillings serve 1 (1 potato)

Ricotta and sun-dried tomato and basil

Snip 3 sun-dried tomatoes (pat dry of any oil if you like) into chunks. Tear 3–4 fresh basil leaves into shreds. Mix with 1 tbsp ricotta, season and spoon in.

Chicken tikka, sweetcorn and natural yogurt

Skin a small, ready-cooked tikka-spice chicken breast and chop into chunks. Mix with 2 tbsp natural yogurt, 2 tbsp sweetcorn and 1 chopped spring onion. Season and spoon in.

Mexican salsa (low fat)

Chop 1 medium-sized tomato and $\frac{1}{2}$ small red or green pepper. Mix with $\frac{1}{2}$ tsp mild chilli, $\frac{1}{2}$ tsp ground cumin, 1 chopped spring onion, 1 tsp oil and the juice of $\frac{1}{2}$ lime, then snip in some fresh coriander or parsley. Spoon in. Top with 1 tbsp grated cheddar, if you like, or 2 tbsp canned red kidney beans. Good for Supersizers.

fillings for wraps

The key with wraps is to use quite soft fillings, and the beauty of that is there's no need for butter. Make sure other ingredients are shredded for easy eating. Cut each wrap in 2 or 3 and pack tightly in cling film to help the filling bind. Perfect for packed lunches.

Fillings serve 1 (1 wrap)

Hummus and veggie sticks

Spread 2 tbsp hummus over a wrap and lay spinach or leafy lettuce over the top. Cut a small carrot, 1/4 green pepper, 3cm-chunk cucumber into thin sticks and scatter over. Season and sprinkle with lemon juice, then wrap up tightly.

Rare beef and beetroot

Mix 1 tbsp horseradish relish with 2 tsp reduced-fat crème fraiche and spread over a wrap. Sprinkle with 2 tbsp chopped cooked beetroot and lay over 2 slices rare roast beef (bought from a deli counter). Season with pepper and scatter with salad leaves or rocket and roll up.

Guacamole and prawn

Crush half a small ripe avocado with a fork and mix with a squeeze of fresh lime juice, a pinch or two of cumin and mild chilli powder and a little garlic puree. Spread over the wrap and lay over some baby spinach or leafy lettuce. Pat dry 3–4 tbsp cooked peeled prawns, scatter over and roll up. Remember: avocado may be higher in fat than other vegetables but it is a good healthy monounsaturated fat and has vitamin E and other useful minerals.

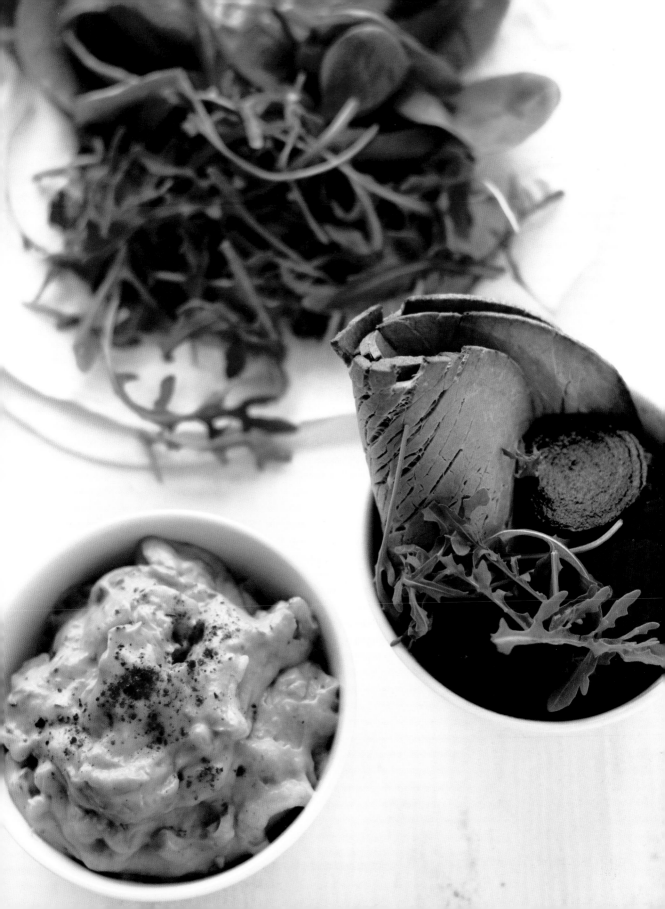

light celery soup

Simple and full of natural flavour, this is a delicious, filling and low-calorie soup.

Serves 4: freeze half

1 head celery, sliced or chopped finely
1 tbsp olive oil
1 onion, chopped
1 sprig fresh thyme
600ml stock, can be made with a cube or bouillon powder
300ml semi-skimmed milk
freshly chopped parsley, to serve

Lean Tip
Oil and water sauté: when sautéing vegetables for soups and stews, adding a little water in this way helps soften the vegetables while they gently fry.

1 Put the celery, onion and oil into a large saucepan with 3 tbsp water. Stir together then heat until sizzling. Reduce the heat, cover and cook for 10 minutes until softened.
2 Add the thyme and stock, season with sea salt and freshly ground black pepper and bring to the boil, then simmer, partially covered, for 15 minutes until softened. Strain off and reserve the stock. Blitz the celery in a blender until smooth, adding back the reserved stock.
3 Return to the pan, stir in the milk and simmer again for 5 minutes. Check the seasoning and serve, sprinkled with parsley.

indian lentil and carrot soup

A great-tasting soup that's quick and easy to make, low in fat and high in protein and carbohydrate.

Serves 4: freeze half

100g red lentils
1 medium-sized onion, chopped finely
2 carrots, grated
1–2 fat cloves garlic, crushed
2 tsp grated fresh root ginger or 1 tbsp ginger puree
1 large fresh green chilli, seeded and thinly sliced, optional
1 tbsp mild curry paste
1.25 litres stock, made with a cube or bouillon powder
a squeeze of fresh lemon juice
2 tbsp reduced-fat crème fraiche (for Superskinnies), to serve
small bunch coriander sprigs, roughly chopped, to serve

1 Put everything from the lentils to the stock into a large saucepan, adding the chilli if you want an extra spicy kick.
2 Season with sea salt and freshly ground black pepper and bring to the boil, stirring, then turn down to a gentle simmer and cook, uncovered, for 15–20 minutes until thickened.
3 Add a squeeze of lemon juice, then stir in the reduced-fat crème fraiche (if using; don't add before freezing) until blended in, and serve topped with coriander.

supersizesuperskinny

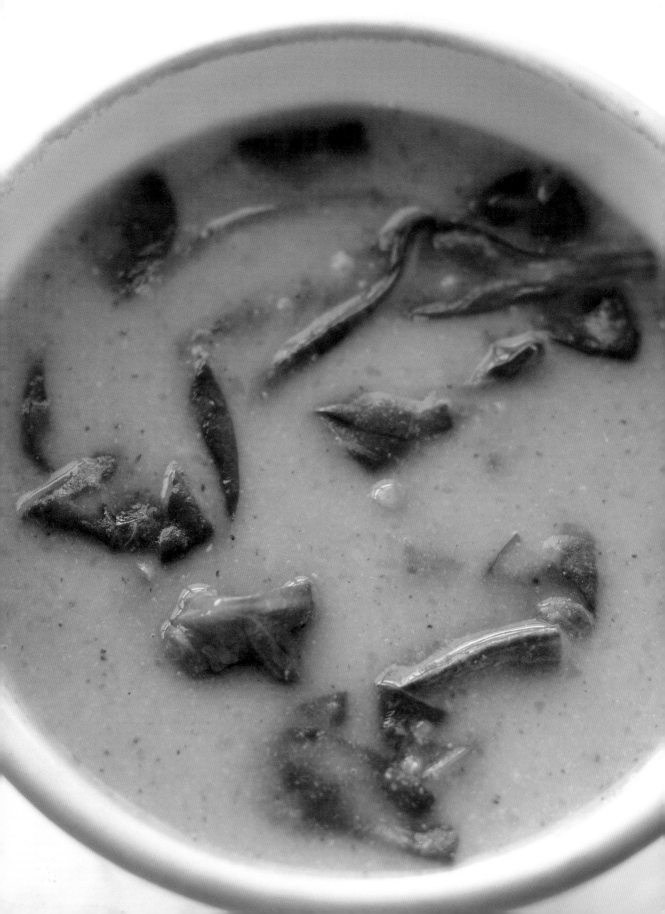

creamy leek, broccoli and spinach soup

Rice adds the creamy texture here – so simple.

Serves 4: freeze half

1 large leek, root trimmed
½ head broccoli, including the thick stalk
1 tbsp olive oil
1 litre stock, made with a cube or bouillon powder
3 tbsp long-grain, basmati or risotto rice (not easy-cook grains)
250ml semi-skimmed milk
a small bag (about 100g) baby leaf spinach

1 Slit the leek lengthways and wash well then slice thinly, including the green ends. Chop the broccoli into fairly small pieces, florets and stalks. Place in a large saucepan with the oil and about 3 tbsp water.
2 Sauté on a medium heat, stirring for about 5 minutes until softened, then pour in the stock and bring to the boil. Stir in the rice, season with sea salt and freshly ground black pepper, lower the heat to a simmer and cook for about 20 minutes until the rice is soft.
3 Remove and strain off the liquid into a jug. Place the vegetables in a blender or food processor and whiz until creamy, gradually adding back the liquid. Return to the pan and mix in the milk, then bring back to a simmer.
4 Drop in the spinach and cook for about 2 minutes until wilted. Check the seasoning and serve.

supersizesuperskinny

smoked haddock, corn and tomato chowder

A main-meal soup. Great with a chunk of crusty bread.

Serves 2

1 medium-sized onion, diced
1 medium-sized potato, peeled and diced
1 stick celery, diced
½ green pepper, seeded and diced
1 scant tbsp olive oil
500ml stock, made with a cube or bouillon powder
1 fillet undyed smoked haddock, about 200g
1 x 200g can sweetcorn, drained
1 large tomato, chopped
200ml semi-skimmed milk
freshly chopped parsley, to serve

1 Put the onion, potato, celery and pepper into a large saucepan with the oil and about 3 tbsp water. Heat until sizzling, stir, cover with a lid and cook on a medium heat for about 5 minutes.
2 Stir in the stock, bring to the boil then reduce the heat and simmer, uncovered, for 12–15 minutes until the potato is softened and has thickened the stock.
3 Skin the fish by running a sharp long-bladed knife between the flesh and skin, then check for any bones. Break up the flesh into small pieces and drop into the simmering stock with the corn and tomato. Stir in the milk.
4 Return to a simmer and cook for another 5–7 minutes until the fish is cooked then check the seasoning and serve sprinkled with parsley.

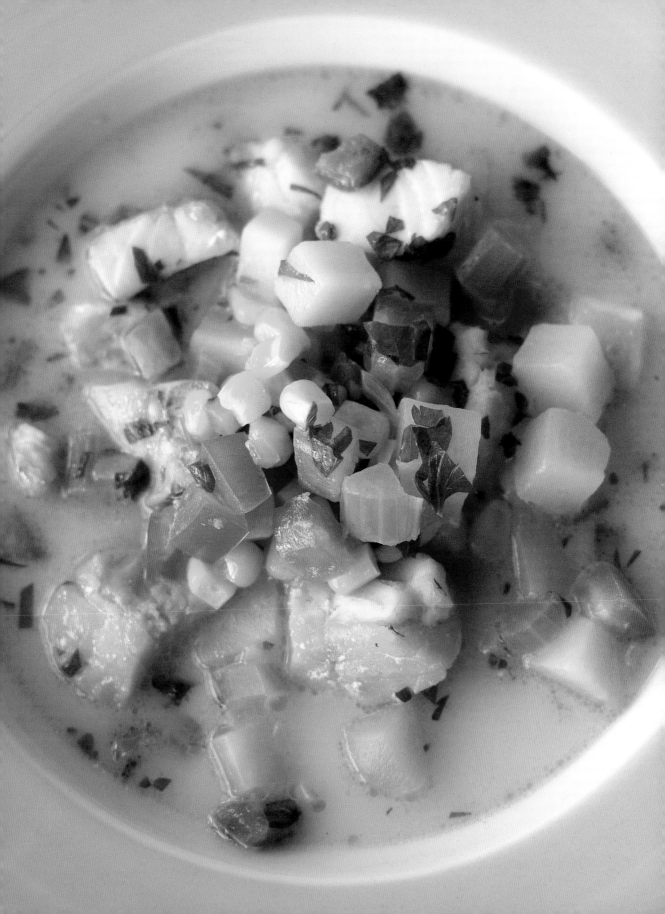

pumpkin and bacon soup

Use a bread knife to cut the pumpkin into large chunks. You don't have to peel it, but if you want to, or the skin looks very thick, use a sharp vegetable knife to do so. Then cut the chunks into small pieces.

Serves 4: freeze half

wedge of fresh pumpkin, about 750g,
    deseeded and chopped into small pieces
1 onion, chopped
1 fat clove garlic, crushed
1 tbsp olive oil
½ tsp mild curry powder
about 100ml dry cider, optional
1 litre stock, made with a cube or bouillon powder
2 tbsp freshly grated parmesan cheese
2 tbsp reduced-fat crème fraiche, to serve (for Superskinnies)
4–6 rashers lean streaky bacon or pancetta, to serve

1 Place the pumpkin in a large saucepan with the onion, garlic, oil and 3 tbsp water. Heat until sizzling then cover and cook on a lower heat for 5 minutes until softened.

2 Stir in the curry powder, then the cider, if using. Cook until the cider evaporates, season with sea salt and freshly ground black pepper and add the stock. Bring to the boil and simmer for about 15 minutes until the flesh is soft.

3 Strain off the liquid and reserve. Whiz the flesh in a blender or food processor with the parmesan, if using, then pour in the reserved liquid and return to the pan.

4 Check the seasoning and whisk in the crème fraiche, if using. Set aside while you grill the bacon until crisp and crinkly. Drain on paper towel and break into chunks. Serve sprinkled on the top of the soup.

lean-line lasagne

Homemade lasagne will have a lower saturated-fat level than a shop-bought one. Use the ragu sauce from page 181. To save time, you could use no-cook or fresh pasta sheets. To vary the dish, thinly slice a courgette lengthways (use a vegetable peeler) and layer it in with the sauce and the pasta.

Serves 2

1/2 ragu bolognese sauce (see page 181)
4 lasagne pasta sheets
40g freshly grated parmesan cheese
1 tomato, sliced
Sauce
300ml semi-skimmed milk
1 tsp olive oil spread
2 tbsp flour
a little freshly grated nutmeg

1 Make the ragu and use half. If using frozen, ensure it is well thawed.
2 Heat the oven to 190°C/Gas 5. Boil the pasta sheets in salted water for 2–3 minutes until softened, unless using no-cook sheets. Drain and slip into a large bowl of cold water.
3 Make the sauce: put the milk, spread and flour into a non-stick saucepan and place over a medium heat, stirring briskly until the flour is blended and the sauce thickens. Cook for a few seconds then remove from the heat and season with the nutmeg and sea salt and freshly ground black pepper.
4 Drain the pasta again and pat dry with a clean tea towel. Spoon half the ragu on to the base of an oval dish and drizzle over a third of the sauce. Sprinkle with 1 tbsp cheese and lay 2 sheets of pasta on top. Repeat with the remaining ragu, another third of sauce and cheese, and the remaining pasta sheets.
5 Drizzle the final third of sauce on top, scatter with the tomato slices and cover with the last of the cheese. Bake for 15–20 minutes until bubbling and browned on top. Cool for a good 10 minutes so the dish firms slightly for easier serving.

tagliatelle with prawns, parsley and chilli

A fabulously easy dinner. As a variation, use the meat from a medium-sized freshly dressed crab in place of the prawns.

Serves 2

125g tagliatelle or linguine

½ tbsp or 1 spritz olive oil

150g peeled prawns, thawed if frozen

1–2 fat cloves garlic, crushed

1 large fresh red chilli, seeded and thinly sliced

2–3 tbsp dry white wine or dry vermouth

a small mugful of fresh parsley leaves, ideally flat-leaf,
    roughly snipped with scissors

2 lemon quarters, to serve

1 Put the pasta on to boil in a large pan with about 1.5 litres lightly salted water. Cook according to pack instructions.

2 Meanwhile, heat a large non-stick frying pan or wok, add the oil and stir-fry the prawns, garlic and chilli for 1–2 minutes. Stir in the wine or vermouth and cook until bubbling, then toss in the parsley.

3 Drain the pasta, leaving it slightly wet, and immediately mix into the prawns. Check the seasoning and divide between 2 shallow bowls. Serve with the lemon quarters alongside to squeeze over.

easy pea and ham risotto

Traditional risotto needs constant stirring for a good 20 minutes, but you can take a shortcut by precooking the rice and then mixing it with a sauce for almost the same creamy texture.

Serves 2

150g risotto rice, such as arborio, carnaroli, vialone nano
600ml stock, made with a cube or bouillon powder
1/2 tbsp or 1 spritz olive oil
1 medium-sized onion, chopped
1 fat clove garlic, crushed
125g frozen peas, thawed
2 slices ham, cut in small pieces
3 tbsp freshly grated parmesan cheese

1 Cook the rice gently in the stock in a large pan for 15 minutes until the grains are just tender. Do not drain.
2 Meanwhile, heat a frying pan until hot, add the oil and sauté the onion and garlic for 5 minutes, then mix in the peas and ham and stir-fry for 2–3 more minutes.
3 Stir the peas and ham into the cooked risotto with half the cheese and check the seasoning. Divide between 2 shallow bowls and serve sprinkled with the remaining cheese.

big spicy chicken salad

Make this dish your template for many a delicious main meal. Take a big plateful of mixed salad leaves of your choice and add a healthy and filling main-meal ingredient such as chicken, fish, prawns, steak or tofu. Top with other salad vegetables such as peppers, carrot strips, tomatoes and lentil sprouts (to grow your own, see below), then add crunch with a seed mixture and accompany with boiled baby new or baked potatoes.

Serves 2

2 skinless, boneless chicken breasts, about 125g each

$\frac{1}{2}$ tbsp olive oil

1 tsp mild curry or Thai or Mexican spice mix

dried thyme or oregano

large bag of mixed salad leaves

1 small carrot, coarsely grated or cut in wafer-thin strips

$\frac{1}{2}$ red pepper, seeded and thinly sliced

$\frac{1}{4}$ cucumber, thinly sliced, or 75g whole green beans or asparagus tips, blanched and cooled

low-fat vinaigrette, spritzed as needed (see page 166)

1–2 tomatoes, cut in chunks

3–4 tbsp lentil or bean sprouts

1 tbsp mixed seeds, such as sunflower, pumpkin, hemp, sesame

Lean Tip
Grow your own sprouts at home from packs of dried pulses. Soak 2–3 tbsp a time in warm water overnight, then drain and shake into a sprouting tray or large screw-top jar. Place on a semi-sunny windowsill (if using a jar, lie it on its side with the seeds in a line). Rinse and drain twice a day until sprouts appear and grow to around 2cm length. Then enjoy the delicious and super-healthy result.

1 Heat a grill until hot. Brush the chicken with oil. Mix together the spice of your choice, a pinch of dried herb and 1 tsp sea salt then sprinkle this on both sides of the chicken. Grill for 3–5 minutes each side until the flesh feels just firm but not overcooked and dry. Remove and let stand for 5 minutes, then slice into 5 or 6 pieces.

2 Meanwhile, mix together the leaves, carrot, pepper and cucumber, green beans or asparagus. Divide between 2 large plates and spritz with vinaigrette. Arrange tomato chunks around.

3 Put the chicken on top and scatter over the sprouts and seeds.

supersizesuperskinny

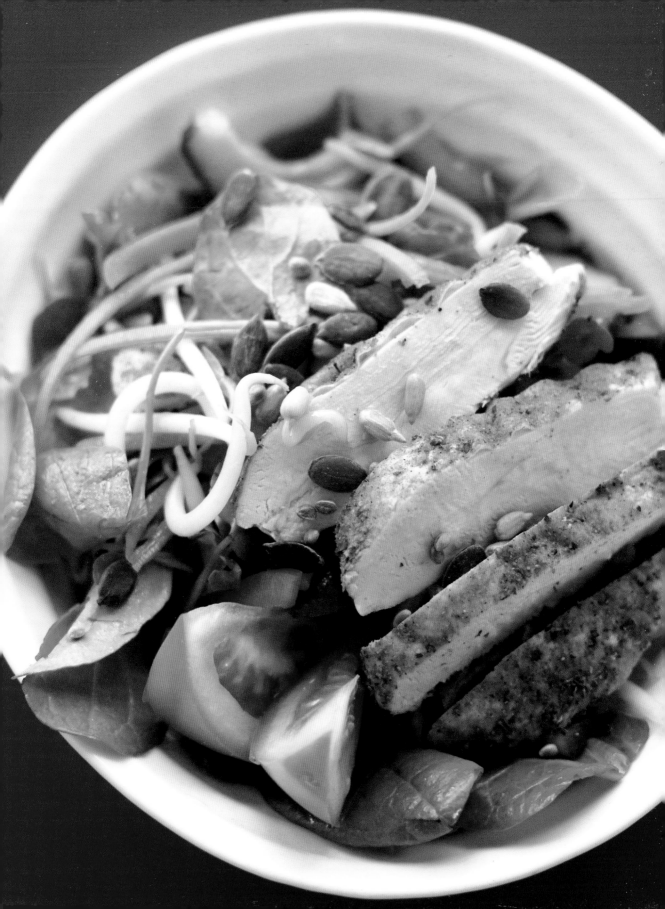

thai green fish curry

Thai curries are great all-in-one meals based on a spicy green broth into which you drop small potatoes and chunks of fish or chicken along with a selection of colourful vegetables. The fresh green paste is whizzed up in a blender – this amount makes double so chill half for another meal. Serve fragrant boiled jasmine rice alongside.

Serves 2

2 tbsp (15g) desiccated coconut

300g new potatoes, halved

250g filleted white fish – such as cod, haddock or monkfish

125g whole green beans, trimmed

6–8 cherry tomatoes

Paste (makes double)

small bunch of fresh coriander (about 25g)

2 large fresh green chillies

3 shallots or 1 medium-sized onion, roughly chopped

2 fat cloves garlic

1 stalk fresh lemon grass, trimmed and roughly chopped

2 Thai kaffir lime leaves, fresh or dried, or grated zest of 1 lime

2–3cm knob of fresh root ginger, roughly chopped

2 tsp ground cumin

1 tsp Thai fish sauce or light soy sauce

juice of 1 lime

1 tbsp vegetable oil

3–4 large fresh basil leaves

1 First make the paste. Pick a good handful of coriander leaves from the bunch and set aside. Roughly chop the remainder and place in a blender with all the other paste ingredients. (If you like a hot curry then simply chop the chillies, otherwise slit and deseed them.) Blend to a thick paste, scraping down the sides once or twice, then scoop half into a large saucepan and the rest into a screw-top jar for the fridge.

2 Mix the coconut with 500ml boiling water and leave to stand for 10 minutes, then strain the liquid into the saucepan and discard the coconut. Add the potatoes and bring to a gentle boil. Simmer for 15 minutes until the potatoes start to soften.

3 Cut the fish into bite-size chunks and add to the potatoes in the pan, along with the beans. Return to simmer and cook for 5 minutes, then add the tomatoes and cook for 2 minutes. Meanwhile, chop the reserved coriander. Divide the curry between 2 dishes, grind black pepper over and scatter the coriander on top.

Chicken curry

Substitute 2 small skinless boneless chicken breasts cut into small cubes and cook for 10 minutes.

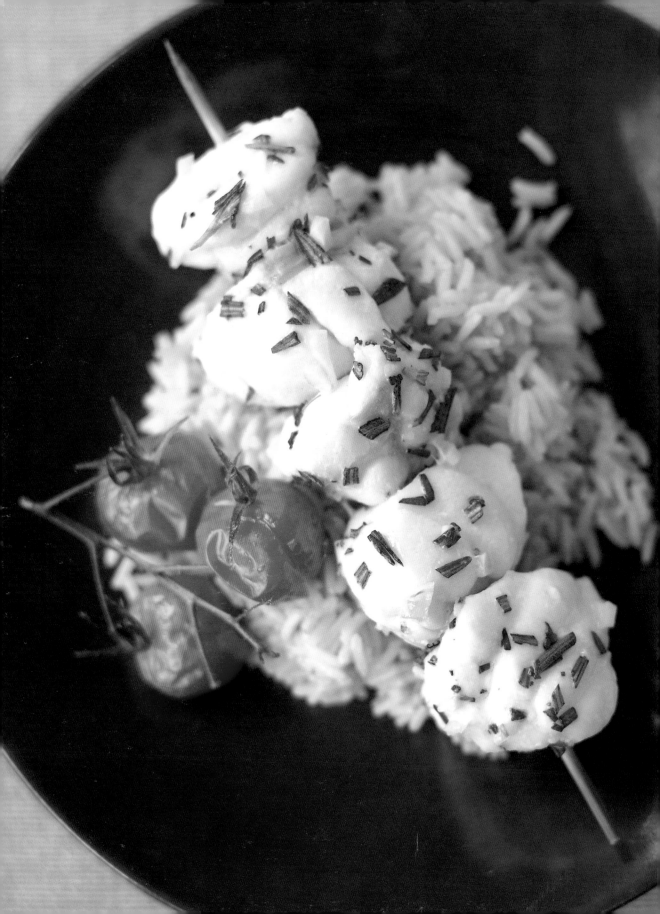

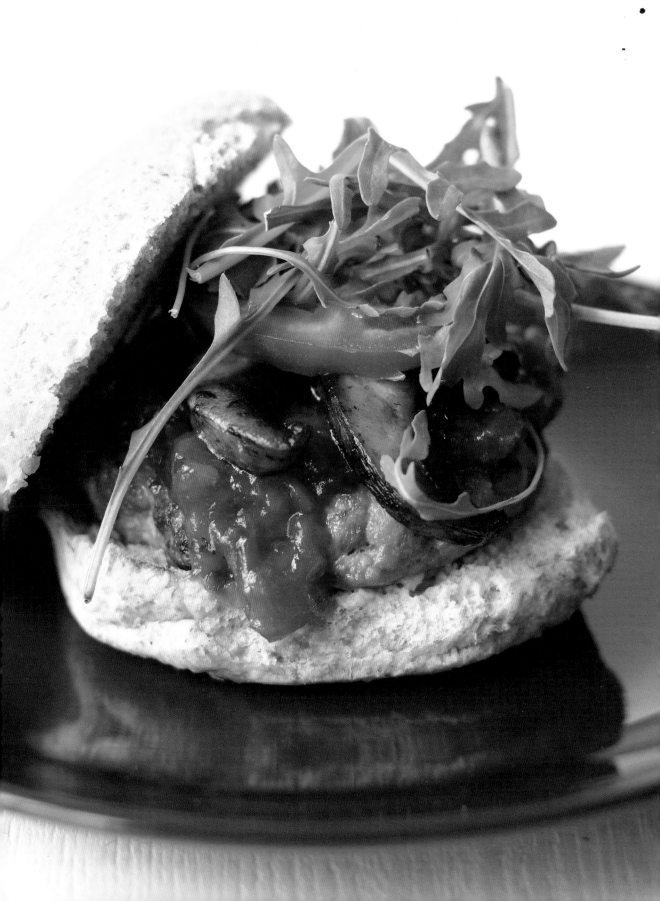

italian steak with tomatoes, peppers and capers

Top grilled steaks with a chunky colourful sauce and serve with tagliatelle or baked potatoes. (You could make double the sauce and freeze half.)

Serves 2

2 trimmed beef or lamb grilling steaks

a little olive oil

leaves of flat-leaf parsley, to serve

Sauce

1 red or yellow pepper, halved, seeded and sliced

1 medium-sized onion, sliced

1 fat clove garlic, crushed

1 tbsp olive oil

1 large beef (marmande) tomato, roughly chopped

a good pinch of dried oregano or thyme

3 anchovies, chopped, optional

2 tsp reduced-fat crème fraiche

1 tbsp capers

1 Make the sauce first. Put the pepper, onion and garlic into a saucepan with the oil and 3 tbsp water. Heat until sizzling, then cover and cook gently for 5 minutes until softened.

2 Stir in the tomato, herbs, anchovies (if using), salt if not using anchovies, and freshly ground black pepper. Cook gently for another 10 minutes until reduced down and pulpy. Mix in the crème fraiche and capers. Set aside.

3 Heat a grill or griddle pan. Brush the steaks lightly each side with oil, season and cook for about 3 minutes each side or until the meat feels lightly springy (i.e. medium).

4 Remove from the heat and stand on a plate for 3 minutes, then spoon over the sauce. Scatter with parsley leaves and serve.

navarin: lamb and spring vegetable casserole

An all-in-one fresh-tasting stew of lean leg-of-lamb chunks and baby spring vegetables.

Serves 2

1 tbsp or 2 spritzes olive oil

250g lean leg of lamb, cut in small chunks

350ml stock, made with a cube or bouillon powder

1 sprig fresh thyme

1 small sprig fresh rosemary

1 medium-sized leek, thinly sliced

4 young thin carrots scrubbed

$\frac{1}{2}$ small fennel, sliced

1 medium-sized turnip, quartered

about 6 new potatoes

a little chopped parsley, to serve

1 Heat a large, heavy-based saucepan, add the oil and brown the lamb. Then pour in the stock, add the herbs and seasoning, cover and simmer gently for about 10 minutes.

2 Uncover and add all the vegetables, including the potatoes. Return to a simmer and cook gently, uncovered, for 15–20 minutes or until the potatoes are soft and the stock reduced by half.

3 Check the seasoning, ladle into 2 shallow bowls and sprinkle with parsley.

supersizesuperskinny

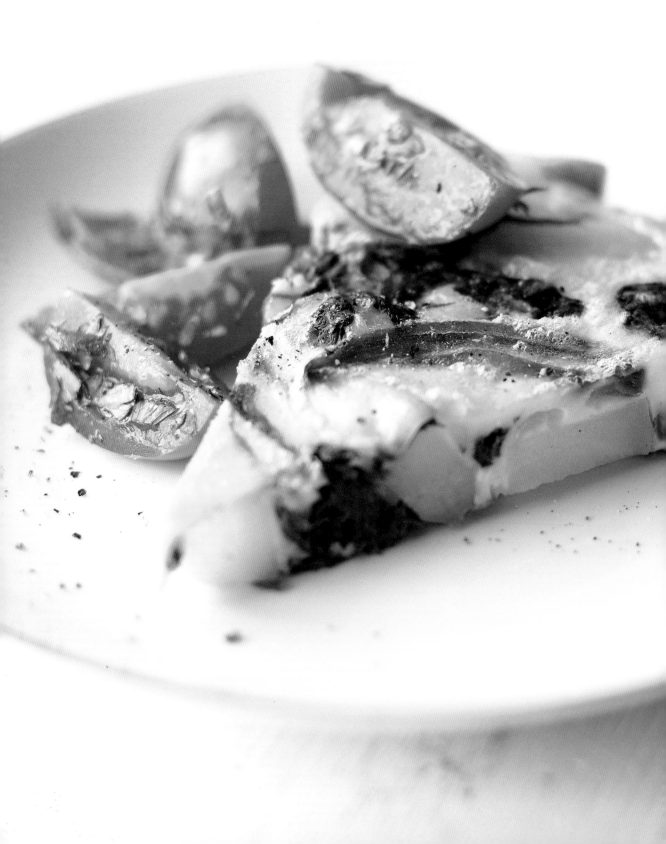

spinach and potato frittata

Turn leftover cooked potato and a bag of spinach into a main-meal omelette. Frittata makes excellent picnic and packed-lunch food. Serve at room temperature or cold, with a tomato salad. Sliced red and yellow peppers, leeks or drained artichokes in jars make good substitutes for the potato or spinach. Meat-eaters might like to slip in slices of parma ham.

Serves 2

1 medium-sized potato or cold cooked potato, about 250g
1 tbsp or 2 spritzes olive oil
1 red onion, sliced
200g bag baby leaf spinach
4 free-range eggs, beaten

1 Peel and cut the potato into chunks then boil for 10 minutes until just tender. Drain. If using leftover potato, simply cut into chunks.
2 Heat a medium-sized non-stick frying pan, add the oil and sauté the onion for 5 minutes until softened, then add the potato chunks and cook for another 5 minutes.
3 Drop in the spinach and stir-fry in the pan until just wilted.
4 Pour in the beaten eggs and swirl in the pan to mix. Season and cook the eggs until they firm, shaking the pan once or twice. When set on top, loosen the sides of the omelette and slide on to a board. Cut into quarters and serve.

moroccan chicken with chickpeas

A warming slow-cook casserole is always welcome, especially if it can be cooked ahead and chilled or frozen ready for reheating.

Serves 2

2 large or 4 small skinless, boneless chicken thighs, cut in chunks
1 medium-sized onion, chopped
1 fat clove garlic, crushed
1 tbsp or 2 spritzes olive oil
½ to 1 tsp chilli powder
a good pinch crushed saffron strands, optional
1 tsp ground cumin
1 small stick cinnamon
1 x 200g can chopped tomatoes
1 courgette, sliced thickly
½ x 400g can chickpeas, drained
juice of ½ lemon
small bunch of coriander, coarsely chopped

1 Sauté the chicken pieces with the onion and garlic in the oil in a large heavy-based saucepan, stirring until browned.
2 Sprinkle in the spices and cook for 5 minutes, then add the tomatoes and courgette, and season with salt and freshly ground black pepper. Cover and simmer for 20 minutes, stirring once or twice.
3 Add the chickpeas and lemon juice and cook for 5 minutes. Check the seasoning and sprinkle with the coriander to serve.

Quick couscous
Cover 125g couscous grains with 300ml boiling water and mix in 1 tsp ground paprika and seasoning. Cool, stirring briskly with a fork two or three times as the grains swell, then leave until cold. Mix in ½ red pepper, finely chopped, and a chopped medium-sized tomato. Reheat in a microwave until piping hot. Or try the Inca super-grain quinoa as an alternative to couscous.

supersizesuperskinny

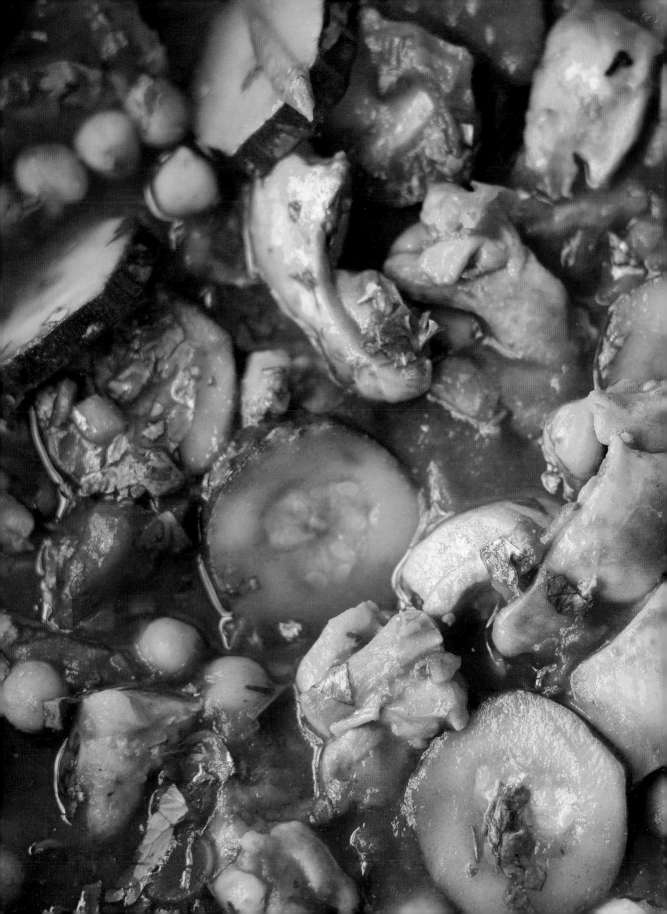

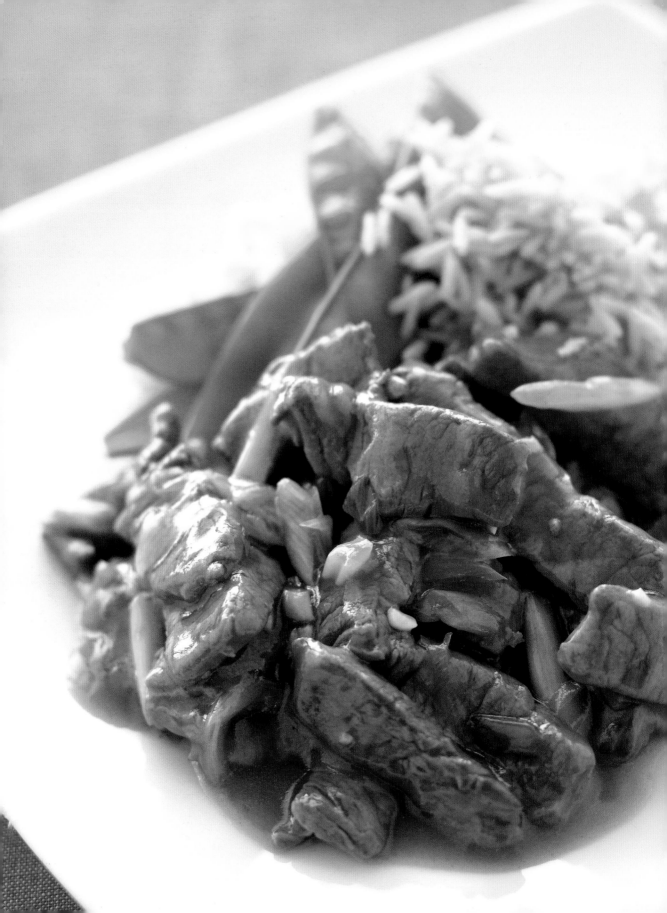

beef stir-fry with oyster sauce

Serve with microwaved mangetouts or bok choi and plain boiled rice, ideally brown basmati.

Serves 2

250g beefsteak, such as sirloin or rump, thinly sliced

1/2 tbsp vegetable oil

1 tsp sesame oil

1 tbsp grated fresh root ginger or ginger puree

1 clove garlic, crushed

1 tbsp oyster sauce

1 tbsp dry sherry, optional

2 tsp cornflour

2 spring onions, shredded

small bunch of fresh coriander leaves, optional

1 Marinate the beef with the oils, ginger and garlic for 10 minutes.

2 Mix together the oyster sauce, sherry and cornflour in a cup with 4 tbsp cold water and some black pepper.

3 Heat a non-stick wok over a high heat, toss in the steak and stir-fry quickly for about 2 minutes. Add the onions and cook for 1 minute.

4 Pour in the oyster sauce mix and stir quickly until thickened, then remove from the heat, check the seasoning and serve, with the coriander leaves, if using, scattered on top.

ham, pepper and pineapple stir-fry

A new variation on the retro combination of grilled gammon and pineapple.
Serve with oven chips or baked potato and green beans.

Serves 2

1 tbsp or 2 spritzes vegetable oil
1 small green pepper, seeded and sliced
1 small red onion, thinly sliced
1 fresh red chilli, seeded and thinly sliced, optional
1 gammon steak, about 200g, cut in strips
1 tbsp soy sauce
2 rings or 75g fresh pineapple, chopped
small bunch of flat-leaf parsley leaves

1 Heat a wok until hot, then add the oil, pepper, onion, chilli and 3 tbsp water. Stir-fry on a medium heat for 5 minutes, until just softened.
2 Add the gammon strips and stir-fry for 3 minutes until just cooked. Mix in the soy sauce, then the pineapple. Cook for 1 minute, then toss in the parsley, season with black pepper and serve at once.

chilli squid and prawn stir-fry

Ready-prepared squid rings and peeled tiger prawns make this stir-fry fast and furious. Serve with salad – rocket is excellent – and boiled rice.

Serves 2

1 tbsp or 2 spritzes vegetable oil
125g squid rings
150g raw tiger prawns
1 fresh red chilli, seeded and sliced
1 fat clove garlic, thinly sliced
3 spring onions, shredded
2 tbsp sweet chilli sauce
1 tbsp soy sauce
1 lime, halved

1 Heat a wok until hot, add the oil and toss in the seafood, chilli, garlic and onions, stirring for 2 minutes until firm and cooked.
2 Drizzle over the chilli and soy sauces then season with black pepper and tip out immediately on to plates. Squeeze over the lime and serve at once.

old-fashioned meat loaf with tomato and corn salsa

Easy, inexpensive meat loaf is one of the best-loved comfort foods of all time. Serve it hot with the tomato and corn salsa, pasta or mashed potato, then eat the remainder cold, thinly sliced for a packed lunch with salad and baked potato.
Serves 4

The loaf

1 medium slice white bread,
   crusts removed
400g lean beef mince
1 small onion, coarsely grated
1 fat clove garlic, crushed
1–2 tbsp Worcestershire sauce
½ tsp dried mixed herbs or thyme
3 rashers lean back bacon, optional
a little oil, for greasing

Tomato and corn salsa

2 juicy tomatoes, chopped
½ small red onion, chopped
3 tbsp sweetcorn kernels
1 small clove garlic, crushed
1 fresh green chilli, seeded
   and finely chopped, optional
1 tbsp wine vinegar
   (red or white or balsamic)
2 tbsp chopped fresh coriander
   or parsley

1 Dunk the bread in a bowl of cold water for a few seconds, then remove and gently squeeze out excess water. Place in a bowl and break it up with a fork.

2 Mix in the mince, onion, garlic, Worcestershire sauce, herbs, 1 tsp sea salt and freshly ground back pepper to taste.

3 Heat the oven to 180°C/Gas 4. Use either a 500g non-stick loaf tin or plenty of slightly oiled foil. If using a tin, line with the bacon rashers across the width of the tin, allowing them to overlap inside the tin and to hang over the edge. Fill with the mixture, fold the ends of the bacon over the top and cover with tin foil. If using a large sheet of foil, lay out the bacon rashers, slightly overlapping, in the centre. Heap the meat mixture on top in a thick roll, then fold over the bacon, bring the foil up and scrunch to seal, and place in a shallow roasting tin. Bake for 35 minutes, until the meat feels firm when pressed.

4 Make the salsa: mix everything together, seasoning to taste, and leave to marinate for about 20 minutes before serving.

5 Let the freshly cooked loaf stand for 10 minutes, then unwrap, reserving any juices, and cut half into thick slices. Serve with the juices trickled over. The remaining loaf can be chilled and saved for later.

pork vindaloo with raita

Vindaloo is a hot and sour Portuguese-Indian curry dish. How much chilli you use depends on personal taste and heat resistance. Serve with a cooling raita (see page 197) and plain brown basmati rice (see page 195).

Serves 4: freeze half

1 pork tenderloin, about 250g, sliced

Paste

3–4 fresh red chillies, to taste, chopped

1 small onion, roughly chopped

1 tbsp or 2 spritzes vegetable oil

1 tsp lightly crushed black peppercorns

1 1/2 tsp whole cloves

1/2 cinnamon stick, broken

1 tsp cumin seeds

2cm cube fresh root ginger

2 fat cloves garlic, roughly chopped

juice of 1 lemon

1 tsp light soft brown sugar

2 tbsp white wine vinegar

1 For the paste, stir-fry the chillies and onion in the oil in a small frying pan for 2 minutes, then remove and tip into a small blender or food processor. Add the remaining ingredients and whiz to a paste.

2 Heat a non-stick frying pan or wok until hot, then dry-fry the pork pieces for a minute or so on each side until browned. Spoon the paste into the pan and mix in 400ml cold water.

3 Bring to the boil then turn the heat to a simmer, season with a little salt and simmer gently for about 30 minutes until the pork is tender.

supersizesuperskinny

retro korma cottage pie

Give this family favourite a retro seventies twist with mild curry spice, and mix the vegetables for a creamy topping.

Serves 2

250g lean beef or turkey or lamb mince
1 onion, chopped
1 fat clove garlic, crushed
1 tbsp chopped fresh ginger or ginger puree
1 small carrot, coarsely grated
2 tsp mild curry powder
2 sprigs fresh thyme
1 tbsp wholemeal flour
1 tbsp milk powder or desiccated coconut
300ml stock, made with a cube or bouillon powder
125g garden peas

Topping
1 large potato, about 400g, peeled and chopped
1 small swede, peeled and chopped
a little milk, for mashing
2 tbsp flaked almonds (for Superskinnies)

1 For the base, dry-fry the mince in a large non-stick frying pan, stirring the meat until it is in crumbs. Then mix in the onion, garlic, ginger and carrot plus 3–4 tbsp water, and cook until the vegetables have softened.
2 Mix in the curry powder. Strip the leaves from one of the herb sprigs and add to the meat along with the flour and milk powder or coconut, followed by the stock and seasoning to taste. Simmer for a good 12–15 minutes until reduced by half.
3 Meanwhile, cook the potato and swede in salted boiling water for 10–12 minutes until soft, then drain and mash, adding milk until smooth and creamy. Season with freshly ground black pepper.
4 Add the peas to the frying pan and simmer for 2–3 minutes, then tip the mince mixture into a shallow pie dish. Dollop the potato and swede mash on top, and spread with a fork to cover, roughing up the top and scattering with the almonds, if using.
5 Heat a grill pan until hot and brown the top lightly. Serve garnished with the remaining sprig of thyme snipped into pieces.

quorn with ginger, chilli and leeks

A meal without meat or fish that's still high in protein; good with rice or noodles. Instead of quorn, you could use firm smoked tofu.

Serves 2

150g quorn pieces
1 tbsp soy sauce
2 tsp dry sherry or vermouth
1 tsp honey
100ml vegetable stock, made with a cube or bouillon powder
1 tsp cornflour
1 tbsp or 2 spritzes olive oil
1 medium-sized leek, thinly sliced
1 red chilli, seeded and sliced
1 tbsp grated fresh root ginger
a bunch of lentil or bean sprouts (see page 190 for grow-your-own)

1 Mix together the quorn, soy, sherry and honey.
2 Blend the stock with the cornflour.
3 Heat a non-stick wok and swirl or spritz in the oil, then toss in the leek, chilli and ginger. Cook for 2 minutes until just softened.
4 Pour off the marinade from the quorn into the stock, then toss the quorn into the wok for 2 minutes.
5 Stir the stock again and mix quickly into the wok, stirring until it thickens. Season with freshly ground black pepper.
6 Check the seasoning and serve sprinkled with the sprouts.

caponata

Lovers of Italian food will enjoy this Sicilian 'ratatouille' of Mediterranean vegetables in a light, lemony, sweet-sour sauce. Serve it with couscous, brown basmati rice or even small pasta shells, adding chickpeas or serving with grilled lean meat for protein. Make double quantities and store for 2–3 days for another meal.
Serves 4

1 tbsp or 2 spritzes olive oil

1 medium-sized red onion, sliced

2 fillets anchovy, rinsed and dried, then chopped

1 small aubergine, cubed

1 small bulb fennel, halved and sliced or 2 sticks celery, sliced

1 small red and 1 yellow pepper, halved, seeded, and cut into chunks

heart of 1 large globe artichoke (see below)

4 medium-sized vine tomatoes, chopped

1 tbsp tomato paste

2 tsp capers

2 tbsp sultanas

juice of 1 lemon

2 tsp sugar

fresh basil and mint leaves, roughly chopped

1 Heat a large saucepan, add the oil and sauté the onion over medium heat for 5 minutes. Then add the anchovy and cook for 1–2 more minutes until it dissolves.

2 Toss in all the other ingredients except the fresh herbs. Add a mugful of water, some seasoning and bring to the boil, then reduce to a simmer and cook gently, uncovered, for about 20 minutes until the vegetables have softened. Check the seasoning.

3 Set aside briefly to allow the flavours to mellow; aim to serve cool or warm, rather than hot. Scatter with the herbs and serve.

To prepare a globe artichoke
Break off the stem as near the base as possible. Then pull off all the spiky leaves until you get to the hairy choke on top of the meaty heart. Cut this off with a sharp knife. Wash the heart and cut it into thick slices or cubes. Toss it with a little lemon juice if not using it immediately.

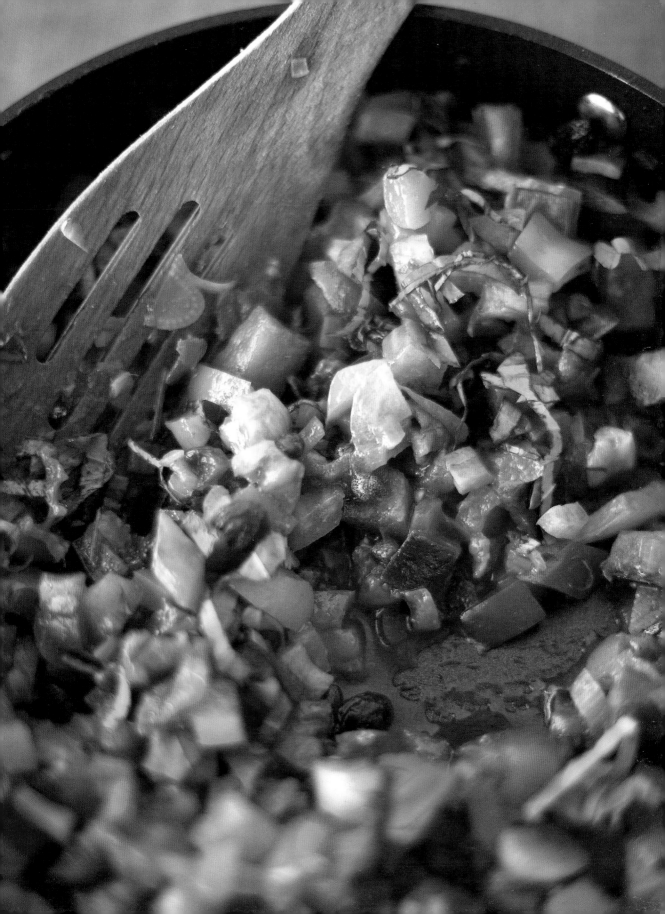

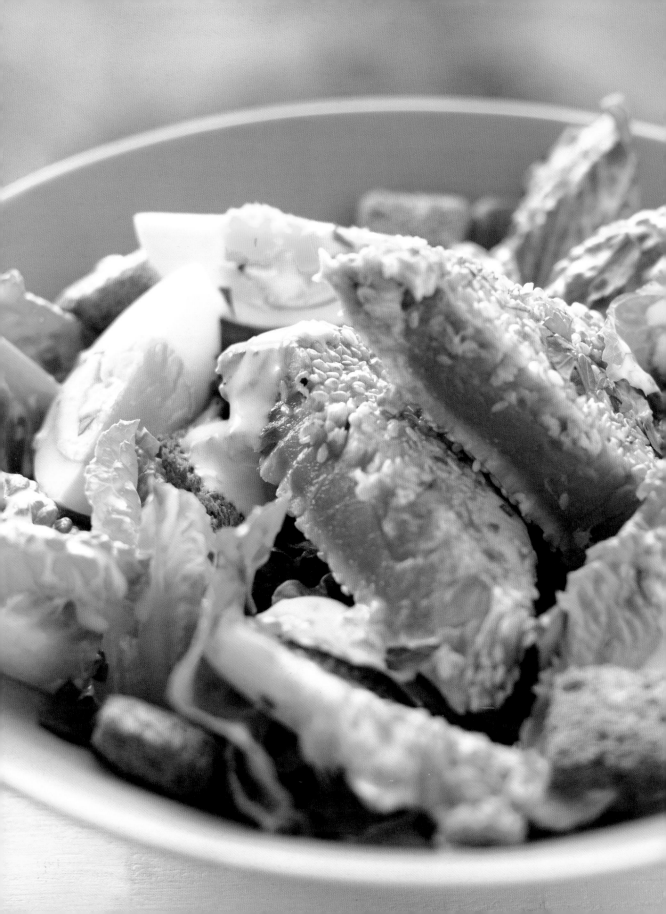

tuna caesar salad

Fresh tuna is lean and meaty, perfect for cooking quickly and tossing into crisp lettuce leaves. The starchy element in this dish comes from home-made croutons. It is the ultimate all-in-one meal.

Serves 2

2 slices wholemeal or brown bread, crusts removed and cut in squares
1 small cos lettuce, torn into bite-size pieces
6 anchovy fillets, rinsed and patted dry
2 tsp mayonnaise
2 small fresh tuna fillets, about 75–100g each, or 1 larger one at 150–200g
1 tbsp sesame seeds
1 medium free-range egg, hard-boiled and quartered, or 2 small tomatoes, quartered
a bunch of flat-leaf parsley sprigs

1 Heat the oven to 180°C/Gas 4. Lay the bread squares on a baking sheet and bake until crisp, about 12–15 minutes. Remove and set aside.
2 Put the lettuce in a bowl. Mash 2 anchovies with the mayo, then gradually mix in 2 tbsp cold water.
3 Sprinkle both sides of the tuna steaks with the sesame seeds and press firmly. Heat a non-stick frying pan or griddle until hot and cook the tuna for about 2 minutes each side if you like tuna pink and springy, a little more if you prefer it firm. Remove and rest 3 minutes.
4 Divide the leaves and the bread cubes between 2 shallow bowls. Slit the remaining anchovies in half lengthways and scatter over, then arrange a tuna steak on top and 2 egg quarters each on the side. Finally, drizzle with the mayo, season with pepper and scatter with parsley. Serve immediately.

filo apple strudel

Ready-rolled filo pastry and dessert apples make it easy to prepare a light version of this well-loved dessert.

Makes 6 slices

2 dessert apples, e.g. Braeburn, Pink Lady etc., peeled

40g dried fruit, such as raisins, dried cranberries, sultanas

2 tbsp (20g) ground almonds

1/2 tsp ground cinnamon

grated zest of 1 lemon

100g filo or about 6 sheets

40g butter (for Superskinnies) or reduced-fat olive oil spread
    (for Supersizers), melted

1 tsp icing sugar

1 Core and chop the apples into small pieces, then toss with the dried fruit, almonds, cinnamon and lemon zest.

2 Heat the oven to 200°C/Gas 6 and cover a baking sheet with a sheet of baking parchment.

3 On the baking sheet, make a layer of filo about 28 x 30cm (probably using 2 sheets; depends on the dimensions of the filo) and brush lightly with butter. Put 2 more layers of pastry on top, brushing lightly in between. Then tip the apple mix down the centre in a neat line. Fold one long edge over the fruit and roll towards the other edge, fully enclosing the fruit.

4 Pull the roll back into the centre of the sheet and brush the last of the butter over the top. Bake for 20–25 minutes until golden and crisp and the apple inside is tender when pierced with a skewer.

5 Remove to a cooling rack until cold, then dust with sifted icing sugar to serve. Cut into portions with a serrated knife.

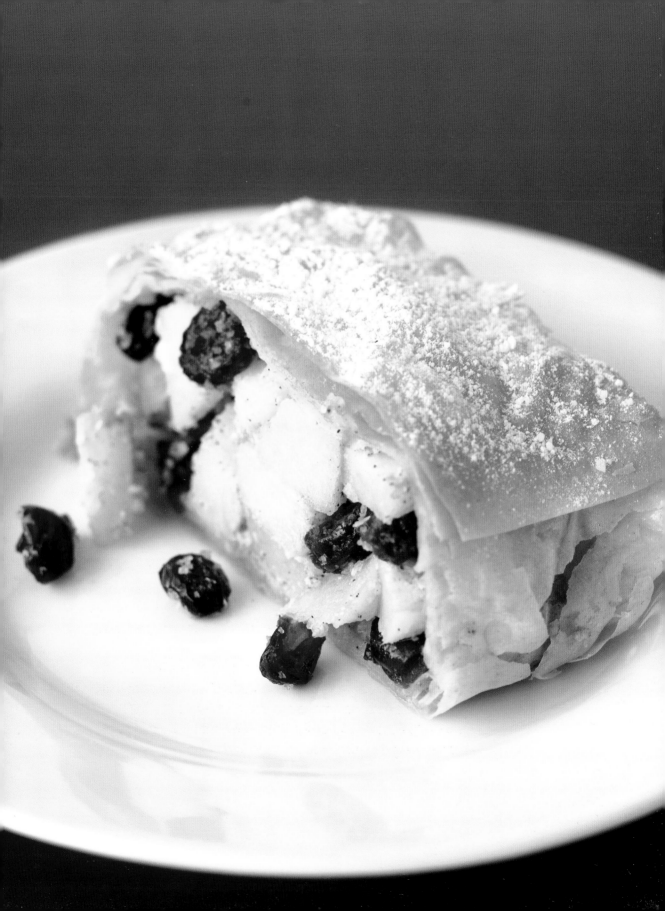

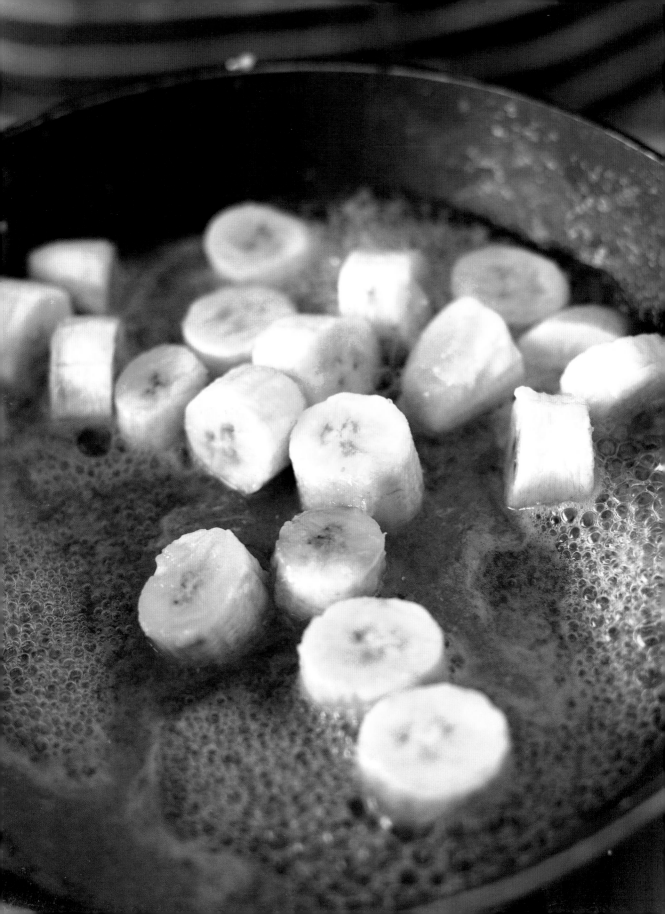

hot bananas with orange and rum

If there are any bananas still in the fruit bowl at the end of the week, this is a great way to use them up and make space for 'restocking'.

Serves 2

2 ripe bananas

1 small orange or clementine, squeezed

2 tsp rum or brandy

2 tsp soft brown sugar, optional

2 tsp single cream or reduced-fat crème fraiche, to serve (optional)

1 Cut the bananas into chunks and place in a small frying pan.
2 Squeeze over the orange juice and add the rum or brandy plus the brown sugar, if using.
3 Heat until the pan sizzles, then cook for 5 minutes over a medium heat, turning the bananas carefully to coat in the juices.
4 Divide between 2 dessert bowls and serve on their own or trickled with some single cream or reduced-fat crème fraiche.

thai rice pudding with mango

Make a creamy and fragrant milky pudding in 15 minutes and serve with slices of fresh mango. Use jasmine rice, which is slightly sticky and cooks quicker than traditional pudding rice. Superskinnies can add coconut cream, if they like.

Serves 4

100g jasmine rice
600ml semi-skimmed milk
1 stem fresh lemon grass or 1 bay leaf
1 tbsp caster sugar or to taste
2 tbsp coconut cream (for Superskinnies)
1 ripe mango, peeled, stoned and cut in slices

1 Put the rice and milk in a large non-stick pan with the lemon grass or bay leaf. Bring to the boil then simmer gently, stirring often, for up to 15 minutes until thickened and creamy.

2 Discard the lemon grass or bay. Add sugar to taste, stir in the coconut cream if using, and set aside to cool.

3 Serve in small dishes with the mango on top.

mini fruity bread and butter puddings

A lighter version of the custard-based dessert, perfectly traditional but not so rich. Substitute fresh sliced fresh plums for the prunes if you have them.

Serves 2

2 slices fruit tea bread
2 large prunes, stoned and sliced
1 medium free-range egg
150ml milk
2 tsp demerara sugar
a little freshly grated nutmeg

1 Cut off the bread crusts and cut in quarters. Put the prunes into 2 ramekins with the bread squares on top.

2 Beat together the egg and milk then pour over the bread, squashing the bread down. Leave to soak for 15 minutes while you heat the oven to 180°C/Gas 4.

3 Place the ramekins in a small roasting dish and pour boiling water around them to come halfway up: a bain marie. Sprinkle the tops of the puddings with demerara and nutmeg.

4 Bake for 15–20 minutes until risen and just firm. Remove carefully from the bain marie and serve.

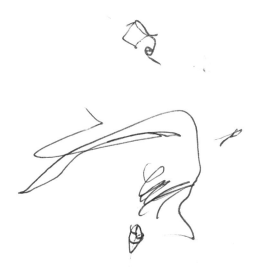

apple and pear crumble

Keep a jar of crumble in the fridge ready to sprinkle over fruit for quick puddings. Add nuts and oats and spices to make it your own special recipe and vary the fruits. It keeps in the fridge for 3–4 weeks. Natural yogurt or reduced-fat crème fraiche is very good with the crumble.

Serves 2, with crumble left over for 6 more servings

Crumble (enough for 8)

50g plain flour

50g wholemeal flour

40g reduced-fat spread or butter

25g porridge oats

1 tbsp demerara sugar

½ tsp mixed spice or cinnamon

1 tbsp desiccated coconut, optional

1½ tbsp chopped roasted hazelnuts or pecans or walnuts, optional

Fruit (enough for 2)

1 large dessert apple, cored and chopped

1 large pear, quartered, cored and chopped

a little pineapple or apple juice, for cooking

1 Whiz together the flours, spread or butter, oats, sugar and cinnamon. Tip into a large jar and mix in the coconut and nuts if using. Store in the fridge until needed.

2 Stew the fruits in just enough juice to cover for about 5 minutes until softened. Heat the oven to 190°C/Gas 5.

3 Tip the fruits into a small pie dish and sprinkle over 4 tbsp crumble (or 2 tbsp per person), then bake for 10–15 minutes until the topping is lightly browned and cooked. Cool and serve.

supersizesuperskinny

In this Extra Helpings section, I compare three of Britain's most popular dishes for various occasions. Now you well know the Gillian McKeith way – to stay healthy you need to eat healthy – but on this very rare occasion, I am going to accept that some of you are not perfect all the time and that a few might feel like you want to tuck into one of the extra helping dishes. This is what you need to look out for to make sure you choose the best option for you.

Breakfast

a) Cooked breakfast of fried egg with bacon, mushrooms, tomato, beans and wholegrain toast
TOTAL around 340 kcals

b) Crunchy oat cereal with a splash of milk and Greek yogurt with honey
TOTAL around 570 kcals

c) Skimmed milk café latte with a large blueberry muffin
TOTAL could be as much as 780 kcals

Surprised the English breakfast has the fewest calories? Well, it's true. An English breakfast has a rotten reputation but it doesn't entirely deserve it. Prepared in the right way there's no reason why you can't have it now and again.

Egg – 1 medium, fried

1 medium egg is lower in calories than you might think: about 80. A great source of protein, which is needed for growth and cell repair. Eggs are also a good source of all the B vitamins, plus the fat-soluble vitamin A. Eggs are one of the few dietary sources of vitamin D, which is essential for healthy bone formation.

★ Fry your egg in a good quality non-stick pan with a minimum amount of oil – just 1 tsp should be enough; or, better still, poach or boil instead and save around 30 calories.

Bacon – 1 rasher rindless back bacon

Although I personally don't eat bacon, if you must, then choose rindless back bacon instead of streaky as it is far leaner. Cut off any visible fat before you cook the bacon.

★ Bacon contains a large proportion of salt. A high-salt diet can lead to high blood pressure. One rasher can contain as much as 1g – so keep it to an occasional indulgence.

Portobello mushrooms – 3 large, grilled or baked

Mushrooms are a useful source of B vitamins and essential minerals potassium, selenium, copper and phosphorous. Potassium is a mineral that helps the body maintain normal heart rhythm, fluid balance, and muscle and nerve function.

Tomato – 1 large, grilled or baked

Tomatoes are a good source of vitamin C. They also provide useful amounts of vitamins A and B6, and are a fantastic source of lypocene, which may help protect the body against certain types of cancer.

★ The tomato and mushrooms add up to 2 portions of the recommended 5-a-day fruit and vegetable servings.

Small portion of baked beans

This small portion of baked beans contains fibre, protein and iron. Choose organic beans with no added sugar or sweeteners. They do exist, and there are varieties sweetened with apple juice. They taste fabulous too.

Wholegrain toast

Wholegrain toast is a good source of fibre, carbohydrate and minerals. Avoid spreading with butter as it will add around 50 calories to your breakfast.

Working lunch

a) Minestrone soup with wholemeal bread roll and butter, followed by a banana and a chocolate wafer biscuit
Total around 600 kcals

b) Triple sandwich, ready salted crisps and fruit drink
Total around 810 kcals

c) Pasta and chicken dish, sliced apple and fruit-flavoured water
TOTAL around 910 kcals

The soup might have been the giveaway here: one look at it and you know you've got something tasty and nutritious — but look at all the other things you can eat with it too, and it still came out with the fewest calories.

Minestrone soup

Minestrone soup is made with tomatoes, onions, herbs, assorted vegetables, beans and pasta. A large bowl of soup will help you to feel fuller for longer with relatively few calories. The vegetables are packed with vitamins and minerals; a serving of vegetable soup will also go towards your recommended 5-a-day portions of fruit and vegetables.

Wholemeal bread roll

Brown bread is a good source of carbohydrate and fibre. Favour wholemeal or wholegrain breads over white as they contain more vitamins and fibre.

Small pat of butter

Butter has such a bad reputation because it's high in saturated fats, which are known to increase blood cholesterol and the risk of heart disease, but it's a pure, unrefined product. However, make sure you keep it to minimal amounts. Alternatively, why not do it my way and drizzle a little extra virgin olive oil or hemp oil over your wholemeal bread before serving. Oils are a good source of essential fats.

Banana

Ideally, your lunch should contain fruit and vegetables. They're packed with antioxidants that promote good health and keep you on that 5-a-day habit. ★ A banana is a good source of carbohydrate and potassium. It also contains a special fibre that promotes good digestion.

Chocolate wafer biscuit

233 calories for a four-finger bar: this chocolate snack contains over a third of the calories of this meal so if you really want to lose weight and eat healthily, cut it out altogether.

Family meal

a) Roast beef with roast potatoes, Yorkshire puddings, vegetables and gravy
TOTAL around 640 kcals

b) Sausage and mash with mixed vegetables
TOTAL around 780 kcals

c) Spaghetti bolognese with garlic bread
TOTAL around 810 kcals

Surely not — a roast dinner with all the trimmings and the fewest calories! Well, life is full of surprises and modern myths, and there's no reason why you can't sit down now and then to a hearty Sunday lunch with all the trimmings if you choose wisely.

Roast beef

First up, some roast beef. Like all meats, beef contains saturated fat and having too much can increase the amount of cholesterol in the blood, which increases the chance of developing heart disease, so if you are going to eat it, then keep to a sensible portion size of 115 grams. It's recommended that you should not eat more than 500 grams of red meat a week (see also the rump steak on page 247). Always choose the leanest cuts, such as topside and sirloin. Roast with the fat on to retain the moisture and flavour of the meat, but remove before serving or eating.

Roast potatoes

Now it's a common myth that starchy foods – known as carbohydrates – are fattening. You just need to watch out for the calorie-laden extras used for cooking and serving, because that's what increases the calorie content.
★ If you are roasting potatoes at home, use a minimal amount of unsaturated oil, such as sunflower oil: 2 tbsp should be enough to cook a whole pan of potatoes serving at least 6 people.

Yorkshire puddings

Many people opt for frozen Yorkshire puddings as they are quick and convenient. At just 53 calories each, you can also keep track of your calories. The ones chosen have no additives (read the labels before you buy) and are made with flour, milk, egg and seasoning.

Mixed vegetables – carrots, peas and cauliflower

The vegetables we used in this dish count towards the 5-a-day recommended amount and are full of vitamins, especially vitamin C – which is essential for healthy skin and a good immune system.
★ Vegetables are very low in calories and are best cooked without salt or butter. Ideally, steam them!

Beef gravy

I prefer a delicious onion gravy, but if you are going for the old beef gravy, then drain as much of the fat from the roasting pan as possible. Add a splash of water to loosen the meaty sediment, then use the vegetable cooking water as stock to add flavour. It's as simple as that.
★ Gravy granules tend to be high in salt, flavourings and colours. So if you don't have the confidence to make your own, choose a fresh organic gravy to serve with your meal.

Takeaway

a) Indian: chicken tikka, channa masala, vegetable curry, basmati rice, poppadom, onion relish
TOTAL around 620 kcals

b) Burger: quarter-pounder with cheese and a medium portion of French fries
TOTAL around 840 kcals

c) Pizza: 3 slices of deep-pan pepperoni pizza
TOTAL around 1050 kcals

Yes, it's true, this huge Indian takeaway has come out with the fewest calories, but it's all down to a careful selection process. No matter how much I tell you to eat healthily, I know that some of you just might eat foods that you're better off without. And come Friday night, you reach for the takeaway menu. Just make sure you don't opt for rich, creamy, calorie-laden curries. Ideally, go for mainly vegetable or pulse-based curries, and just a few pieces of lean chicken.

Chicken tikka

Typically, the chicken is marinated in spices and yogurt, then cooked in a very hot tandoor oven, without the need for additional fat. This keeps the chicken low in fat and calories.

★ If you must eat chicken, only buy it from a reputable establishment that uses good quality meat. If your chicken tikka is highly coloured, it could have been made with excessive amounts of food colourings.

Curries

Topping up on vegetable, lentil and pulse curries will add vitamins, minerals and fewer calories to your meal. Vegetable curries are a great way of incorporating vegetables into your meal and will count towards your 5-a-day recommended amount. Keep an eye on your serving quantity though – even vegetable dishes can contain high levels of salt. A high-salt diet can lead to blood pressure problems. Channa masala is made from chickpeas, which contain useful amounts of protein and fibre. Lentil dahls are also good choices, but can be salty.

★ Ask for your meal to be prepared with as little fat as possible. Indian restaurants often use clarified butter – ghee – for cooking and it is very high in saturated fat.

Plain boiled basmati rice

Wholegrain brown rice is a good source of carbohydrate. In a takeaway, wholegrain may not be offered, so go for plain boiled basmati rice, as pilau rice is fried in oil and spices. And keep the portion size small: it should fill around a third of your plate – no more.

Poppadom

1 poppadom fried in oil contains around 40 calories. I can't suggest poppadoms are a healthy choice but if you do have one with your meal, you won't be pushing the calories too high. Stay off the naan breads though – just half a naan bread could cost you over 260 calories.

Onion relish

Raw onions contain very few calories, so feel free to tuck in. A couple of tablespoons of mango chutney can contain around 80 calories. Yogurt dips are sometimes sweetened with sugar and seasoned with salt, so go for natural yogurt.

Pub grub

a) Jacket potato, baked beans and grated cheese
TOTAL around 710 kcals

b) Scampi, chips, salad, peas and tartare sauce
TOTAL around 950 kcals

c) Cheddar cheese ploughman's
TOTAL around 1020 kcals

Coming in with the lowest calories is this feast of a jacket potato with baked beans and grated cheese. Now this is still a high-calorie lunch option, but of the three choices it is the most filling and probably the most nutritious.

Jacket potato

A jacket potato makes a great base for a filling and healthy meal. Potatoes cooked in their skins are a nice source of fibre – which is essential for a healthy digestive tract. They also contain potassium, which helps the body maintain normal heart rhythm, fluid balance, and muscle and nerve function.

★ A medium jacket potato – when eaten with the skin – could contain around half your daily recommended amount of vitamin C. Vitamin C strengthens blood-vessel walls and promotes wound healing and iron absorption.

★ Jacket potatoes are rich in B vitamins, especially B6, which promotes proper nerve function and the synthesis of red blood cells.

Baked beans

Baked beans contain a good amount of protein and fibre and provide vitamins B6, B1 and folic acid. Remember, some varieties of beans are fairly high in salt and the government recommends that everyone reduces their daily salt intake.

Cheddar

There's no getting away from it, cheddar cheese is high in saturated fat. But grated cheddar – or a similar hard cheese – is what you are going to be served in a pub. So, request that your jacket potato and beans is served with just a small sprinkling of cheese. On the plus side, cheese contains B vitamins and calcium, which helps protect against osteoporosis. You may think that you'd be better off with tuna mayonnaise in your jacket potato, but by the time the pub has added a couple of tablespoons of mayonnaise to your portion, you could be looking at a filling containing up to 300 calories.

Salad garnish

Even a small salad garnish will go towards the target of 5-a-day fruit and vegetables, so don't forget to eat it.

Dinner for two

a) Rump steak with potato wedges, broccoli and peas, mushrooms and tomato
TOTAL around 475 kcals

b) Lamb with roasted vegetables and runner beans
TOTAL around 600 kcals

c) Chicken Kiev with Caesar salad and new potatoes
TOTAL around 730 kcals

Surprised that a meal of steak and potato wedges has the fewest calories? Well, appearances can be deceiving, and as it's just a one-off now and again, your waistline should not overly expand.

Rump steak

It's not for everybody but lean rump steak does contain protein and iron. Protein is essential for growth and cell repair, while low iron stores can cause lethargy, fatigue and increased susceptibility to infections. Like all meats, beef contains saturated fat. Having too much saturated fat can increase the amount of cholesterol in the blood, which increases the chance of developing heart disease. Always choose the leanest cuts and remove any visible fat before eating. Grilling is a good low-fat cooking method for steak.

★ Research suggests that you should cut down on eating red meat. It has shown a link between red meat consumption and some cancers. It's recommended that we should not eat more than 500 grams of red meat a week.

Frozen potato wedges

Generally, it's best to go for thick, chunky chips rather than thin fries, because the proportion of fat to potato will be far less. Oven chips usually contain fewer calories than deep-fried chips, but watch out for some varieties as they could add to the calories, fat and salt in your meal. It is best to make your own by tossing thick wedges of skin-on potato with a little oil and then baking in a hot oven until golden.

Broccoli and peas

All green vegetables are packed with vitamins and minerals. Broccoli is a very good source of fibre and vitamins.

★ Always have vegetables with lunch and dinner. Have them for snacks too.

Baked tomato

Tomatoes are full of vitamin C, which is essential for healthy skin and a strong immune system. They also contain lypocene, which is thought to help protect against some cancers. Add to the baking tray with the potatoes for the last 5 minutes of cooking time.

Mushrooms

Mushrooms are a good source of B vitamins and essential minerals potassium, selenium, copper and phosphorous. Grill, bake or boil your mushrooms.

Party food

a) Deli platter: hummus, smoked salmon, parma ham, marinated olives, mozzarella, breadsticks, carrot sticks, tomato salsa
TOTAL around 430 kcals

b) Party platter: cocktail sausages, half scotch egg, small handful honey-roast cashew nuts, smoked salmon roules, party sausage roll, cheddar and pineapple sticks, cucumber, carrot
TOTAL around 610 kcals

c) Traditional British: 2 buffet pork pies, garlic and onion dip, celery and cherry tomatoes
TOTAL up to 850 kcals

Surprised? Yes, the huge deli platter contains the fewest calories, and it really makes the point that more can be less — you just need to choose carefully.

Hummus
Hummus is made from chickpeas, which are a good source of protein and fibre.

Smoked salmon
Salmon is an excellent source of the essential omega 3 fatty acids, which are vital for controlling blood pressure, balancing hormones and promoting healthy skin.
★ Smoked salmon contains high levels of salt due to the curing process. If you are watching your salt intake, switch to poached salmon and still enjoy all the benefits of oily fish without the sodium.

Parma ham

Although I don't eat ham, parma ham is lean and only contains around 21 calories per slice. It has a full flavour, so a little goes a long way.

Marinated olives

Olives are a great source of monounsaturated fats. Marinated olives are packed with flavour, so you're less likely to miss the salted peanuts.

Mozzarella cheese

Mozzarella cheese contains far fewer calories than a high-fat cheese such as cheddar.

★ A 50g portion of mozzarella contains around 129 calories while a 50g portion of cheddar contains 208 calories. Mozzarella cheese is a good source of bone-strengthening calcium and B vitamins.

Breadsticks

At just 22 calories per stick, you can afford to have the occasional breadstick …

Carrots

… but you are best to top up with vegetable sticks instead – they hardly contain any calories, have heaps of vitamins and minerals, and contribute to your 5-a-day recommended quota of fruit and vegetables.

Tomato salsa

Keep away from creamy dips and opt for tomato salsa instead. Tomatoes are a great source of vitamin C – good for the immune system.

Pudding

a) Fresh fruit pavlova – with strawberries, raspberries and blueberries, whipped cream and grated chocolate
TOTAL around 325 kcals

b) Apple pie and crème fraiche
TOTAL around 425 kcals

c) Chocolate cheesecake
TOTAL up to 530 kcals

Pavlova looks fantastic and even an enormous portion still comes out with the fewest calories.

Meringue nest
Now, meringues are high in sugar and you should all be cutting down on sugar, but one nest will still only contribute 5 per cent of your recommended daily amount of carbohydrate and 12 per cent of sugars.

Berries
The berry bonanza of strawberries, raspberries and blueberries is full of antioxidants. Antioxidants work by preventing cell damage caused by free radicals, unstable molecules that are released when the body uses oxygen. They also contain good amounts of vitamin C, essential for boosting immunity and helping wound healing and iron absorption; plus folic acid. The amount of fruit in this dessert would represent 2 portions of your recommended 5-a-day.

Whipped cream
Go easy on cream – whichever type you use – because it is high in saturated fat. Too much saturated fat can lead to obesity and heart disease.

Plain dark organic chocolate
Chocolate is high in both fat and sugar, so make it go further by finely grating it. Better still, use raw cocoa products without all the sugar and other stuff.

Dr Christian Jessen . . .

presents the hit Channel 4 TV series Supersize vs Superskinny. A qualified medical doctor, Christian is passionate about educating the public across all areas of health. In addition to his detailed knowledge of general medicine, he is an expert on HIV and sexual health, and has practised medicine in both Kenya and Uganda.

Christian has seen first hand the effects of a lack of understanding of basic health issues, and he believes that each of us should take responsibility for our own health and wellbeing. To spread this message he writes regularly for a number of magazines including Arena, FHM, Men's Health, GayTimes and AXM, and he contributes articles to many major UK newspapers.

His ability to make complicated medical information accessible and interesting has also made Christian a popular television presenter. As well as Supersize vs Superskinny, he presents Embarrassing Illnesses on Channel 4 and has a regular phone-in slot on The Wright Stuff on Five. Christian currently practises at a clinic in Harley Street.

'Eating well is probably the easiest way for each of us to take control of our own health. I hope this book gives you the tools to get back in shape and pave the way to a healthier, happier future.'

Endemol would like to extend a special thank you to:

Dr Christian Jessen, Gillian McKeith, Walter Iuzzolino, Sara Ramsden, Colette Foster, Iain Dodgeon, Alex Joffe, Oliver Wright, Fin O'Riordan, Claire Morrison, Claire Edwards and the production team. Sarah Emsley, Roz Denny, Mari Roberts, Polly Andrews, Rebecca Jones, Luigi Bonomi, Amanda Preston, Sue Rider, Lynne Garton, Lynn Greenwood, Justine Patterson, Claire Loades, Smith & Gilmour, Rae Langford, Katie Nicholls, Seema Khan and Sian Piddington.